Yin, Yang, Yogini

A Woman's Quest for Balance,
Strength and Inner Peace

A Memoir

Kathryn E. Livingston

YIN, YANG, YOGINI

Copyright © 2014 Kathryn E. Livingston

eISBN: 978-1-62467-182-1
Print ISBN: 978-1-62467-183-8

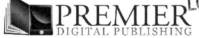

PREMIER
DIGITAL PUBLISHING

Published by Premier Digital Publishing
www.premierdigitalpublishing.com
Follow us on Twitter @PDigitalPub
Follow us on Facebook: Premier Digital Publishing

Author's Note: Other than my immediate family, names and identifying
details of individuals in the following memoir have been changed.

Dedication: For Mitch

"May the pure light within you, guide your way on."

—Irish folk song

Before "The Change"
(AND I DON'T MEAN MENOPAUSE)

By the time you turn fifty, you expect that you'll have everything in order: the socks will all finally be matched and rolled, the refrigerator will be organized with nothing suspicious hiding on the back top shelf, and your career will be stellar. You imagine that the 300 pins that fell out of your sewing box and down the basement stairs when your kids were three, five, and nine and you were way too busy to locate them (the pins, that is) would have been picked up by now. You're done freaking out because you have to color your hair, and you've accepted the fact that you're probably never going to wear a bikini again (or, if you do, your breasts are not going to look quite up to snuff in it).

But that's not what happened to me. For me, fifty was just the *start* of something. Fifty was my turning point, because it was then that I began to realize I didn't want to be me— myself— anymore. Or rather, that I didn't want to be the person I *seemed* to be. I wanted to shed the baggage I'd been carrying for half a century, and start all over. But how to do that?

At fifty I was ten pounds overweight. I was perpetually worried about dying (i.e. a dented can of kidney beans purchased at the grocery store meant rigor mortis would soon set in). Airplanes scared the crap out of me. As did cars. I was obsessed about getting my kids into decent colleges. Negative self talk was rampant: I would lecture myself for hours about what a lousy writer, mother, wife, hiker, cook, swimmer, shopper, dresser, make-up putter-on-er or whatever else I could think of I was.

My mother—my best friend and fellow worrier— had died just two weeks before 9/11. My fifteen-year-old son was about to embark on a trip to Europe, and I myself had not flown in an airplane for more than twenty years. Driving on highways terrified me. I drank inordinate amounts of wine. I was prone to smoking cigarettes. Oh, did I mention I was ten pounds overweight? Well, maybe it was more like fifteen. I couldn't really walk too far because of the closet smoking and "over-drinking" and really, why would I want to? I didn't know what might be lurking around the next corner: a mugger, a rapist, a pile of dog turd? To me, that was kind of what life seemed to be: a rather arduous walk and around every corner there might be skulking some kind of demon—could just be a kid with a skinned knee, could be a kid with a brain hemorrhage.

My life was like that: always looking on the "dark" side. Always imagining the worst. There were reasons for this, of course, and we'll look into them. Everyone has his or her reasons. But it doesn't have to be this way.

I'm sitting, you see, in Lotus position, which means you have to settle yourself on your rear with your spine straight, bend your knees and place your feet on your thighs. This may sound easy, but it's not. Just try it: I dare you! (But try very gently—I don't want to be sued.) That, however, is not the half it.

I am no longer ten or fifteen, or, okay, twenty pounds

overweight. I weigh exactly what I should weigh. I have no negative comments to make about myself (or very few). I rarely think about death, and when I do it's with curiosity and acceptance. I am proud of my children and confident that they will live long, healthy, successful lives (my eldest is now in Mexico, and my middle son spent last semester in Qatar; the youngest—perhaps the bravest— is in college *and* a rock band). I can do a headstand and a handstand, with ease. My life is filled with angelic, compassionate, gentle friends—many of whom I have only met in the past few years. I am not afraid to drive on highways. Airplanes don't scare me. *Cancer* doesn't scare me (not that it excites me, either!)

The answer? Yoga. Yes, yes, I know it's a hackneyed word, bandied about by ancient yogis for thousands of years. And so many are doing it.

But are *you* doing it?

If you *are*, you will understand my story. If you *aren't*, you must read my story. But remember—yoga isn't a quick fix; it seeps into your bones, your heart, and your soul over time.

YEAR ONE

"The body is the temple of the soul."
—B.K.S. Iyengar

"This life is more than just a read through."
—Red Hot Chili Peppers

The Family Jewels

I'm off to yoga today, for the first time in my life. I go blind, deaf and very dumb; not knowing at all what yoga is about. I suspect it might involve a little stretching, and maybe keeping my eyes shut for longer than usual (as in playing Marco Polo at the pool with the kids). I have no idea that people stand on their heads, or maneuver into a "Downward-Facing Dog" posture that makes one feel as if one's skull will burst at the same time one's legs collapse. I'm shocked that each class begins and ends with "Om" in unison, a practice that I find both terrifying and embarrassing.

I've come to yoga class because I'm falling apart. My therapist (a soft-spoken, slender lady whom I've recently begun seeing) believes it might pull me together. I'm doubtful, but what's to lose? I have a wonderful husband, three perfect boys, and a charming, little home in a New Jersey suburb. On the outside, I appear content and in control, but something tugs violently at my heart each morning; the mistakes I've made, the wrong turns

I've taken, the losses that come with middle age, including the deaths of both of my parents. I have yet to find the gains of aging (except at my waist). Might yoga be a path?

I need a path because life has come to a sudden halt, as if I've stubbed my toe at the gate to year fifty, and sit bleeding. I'm afraid to pick myself up and carry on. I'm afraid to move forward, and I can't go back, and in my paralyzed state, I wonder if I'll even be able to figure this yoga thing out at all. In the past, I would have turned to my mother; though she couldn't calm my fears because she had too many of her own, at least we could commiserate. But now she's gone, and there's no one who seems to understand the agitated state of my mind. When I crawl into bed at night, my thoughts take hours to settle, and even when I'm sleeping my worries seem to hum and vibrate beneath my pillow. I'm literally "driving myself crazy," and without my mom in the passenger seat, I know I can't continue to travel through life in this way.

I'm afraid of little things, like traffic merges and snapping turtles, but I'm also afraid of sending my fifteen –year- old son off to study in England for a month, afraid of flying, of losing my three nearly grown boys to adulthood and independence, frightened at the thought of them going off to college, afraid of illness, terrified of death—my own, and everyone else's— and even scared of fully enjoying life because it can so easily slip between one's fingers. I hope—and if I prayed I'd be praying— that yoga will make a difference. But I'm not a spiritual woman, and I'm certainly not an avid exerciser. I haven't been to church in more than twenty years, and the last time I moved fast enough to break a sweat, I was chasing a toddler around a park.

I've decided to give yoga a chance to help me find some kind of solace, imagining that it will be a relaxing pursuit, akin to nibbling a cannoli and sipping cappuccino in the Village on a spring night. Bizarrely enough, a new yoga studio has opened just a block away from my house, and today, I walk there somewhat hopefully, even though my heart beats wildly. There's no way I can know, at this time and place in my life, that yoga will transform me, that it will not only help me to lose those unwanted pounds, but that it will guide me to an unwavering sense of a higher power I'd never dared before believe existed, that it will steer me toward courage, strength and a kind of mental peace I'd never imagined possible. I have no idea that the asanas (or postures), breathing exercises, and yoga sutras (or threads of thought), will turn me from a woman who fears the sound of my very own footsteps, to one who will learn to accept loss and impermanence, will change me into someone who will have the courage to combat a terrifying disease, will help me to become a woman whose doubts and fears will be overcome by the embrace of gratitude, trust, and grace. There's no way I can know that standing on my head will turn my life right-side up, and I can't possibly foresee that the friends and connections I will make in this tiny studio will inspire me to forever alter the way I approach the very things that scare me the most.

No, I can't know any of this at this moment, because my inner journey has just begun.

I open the glass door to the studio and tiptoe inside; a line of shoes greets me in the foyer, and I have the sense to kick off my sandals. The place smells like lavender and spice, and as I round the corner I notice candles burning near a trickling fountain.

"Welcome!" says a small, friendly woman behind a glass desk. "You can grab a mat here."

"I've never practiced before…" I begin softly.

"No problem!" she waves her hand at me. "Just fill this out, please."

I quickly scribble my vitals on a health form, opting not to mention my jumping-bean brain. Inside the yoga room, I place my mat on the floor and lower myself with a thud, glancing nervously at the young, sculpted women all around me. Within moments it's clear that this yoga class has more in common with a rabid tiger than Italian pastries and mellow nights.

The teacher, a striking, big boned woman who introduces herself as "Ali" sits cross-legged at the head of the class. "Hands to your heart," she says sweetly, and then begins to chant "Om" as the other women raise their hands to their chests and chant along. Maybe if I squeeze my eyelids hard enough, I'll wake up and be somewhere else.

Instead, we all rise, lifting our arms above our heads and sending our right legs out behind us. I fall to one side, then the other, knees and muscles as gelatinous as seaweed in a wave. I've always thought of yoga—if I've given it any thought at all—as simply a word, a benign and friendly word like yodel. It never crossed my mind that yoga would involve something called a "lunge," that I'd be required to energetically snap my leg forward, lift up my back heel and balance with my arms upraised.

As I tip and sway, the teacher walks toward me, perhaps surprised to find a novice in her midst. "Your first time?" she whispers in my ear as I struggle. I nod and she smiles, yet I sense just a hint of disapproval.

Ali, gleaming muscles and large, dark eyes, speaks softly as she drives us. She has no mercy for "beginners" like me; in this yoga class we're all treated as equals. I ape the movements (and I do mean ape), unsure of where to put my hands and feet, my arms and legs trembling. I'm astonished by the unfamiliarity of the poses and my body's lack of cooperation, but I press on.

I am here not just because I need an answer, but also because I need a way. It seems that all the love that has guided me my whole life, has finally come into bloom, and in the blooming I have realized how much it hurts to let go, to move on, to say good- bye. Pain can come from happiness, from love, from contentment, as well as from loss and hurt. Pain can come from wanting to keep everything the same forever— an impossible task. And fear…fear can come from things that aren't there and are never going to happen, as easily as from things we can see and touch. This is the kind of fear that has plagued me forever; I want to find a way to put it to rest, a way to quiet the frightened child that seems to have taken up permanent residence in my adult body.

I've been holding back for far too long, closing my eyes and saying, "No." My parents raised me on what my friend Eloise and I call "the Iceberg Theory" of life: we're all standing on a huge cake of ice in a churning ocean, and at any minute the ice may crack. Others will watch—loved ones, friends, even strangers—horrified, as the unfortunate floats out to sea or falls off the slab into the frigid water. Even children can go without warning. The worst part is not knowing: will you and your loved ones get to stay on the slab, or fall off the iceberg prematurely?

If you bring a child up in this manner, it can work two ways: a child can trust and believe that the Iceberg Theory is true, or a child can say to herself, "this is horseshit." And so it was in my family. My sister, Ruthann, fears nothing. Airplanes don't bother her. She never suspected her kids' babysitters of child molesting. She never worries about smashing into a broken-down car while driving in a blinding snow or dying of botulism from a rotten can of tomatoes. But I took everything my mother said at face value. Her threats and warnings weren't wasted on me—every potential terror was duly recorded in my memory, stored away for when I'd become a mother myself. Then I hauled them out— the whole sack of grizzlies—to distribute to my own children, passed down through the generations like cursed family jewels.

Jewels that I no longer want to polish and cherish.

∽

I head out for my second yoga class, still wary and doubtful that I'll ever be able to master even the brainless "Corpse" pose, which involves resting motionless on one's back. Only three people show up tonight. Again, Ali is our teacher. After tonight, she now knows my name. Kathryn: she who burps.

Yoga class is very still. Music plays softly in the background; Indian, New Age, classical. Breath…breathing… the air gliding in and out of our lungs ("through the nose only!") as predictably as the surf. Before class, I had wolfed down a tuna burger and a mound of cabbage. Dinner was late—my fault, since I was attempting to finish reading a novel while grilling the fish— and now I know why the yoga books instruct that a light meal be consumed two hours before class (or three if the meal includes meat): otherwise one might fart or belch one's way through the poses, which would be like coughing during the Queen of the Night's aria in The Magic Flute, or having one's cell phone go off during the overture to Figaro (my husband, Mitch, plays clarinet with the New York City Opera, thus my penchant for musical analogies). For a moment, I fear that my burgeoning yoga life has been forever ruined.

But no one says a word. Not even a snigger. Just the breath; in and out, in and out, slowly. My raucous burp is respectfully ignored in a way it never would have been in seventh grade science class, when *someone* surely would have hooted with wild Medieval belly-laughter, pointing short calloused fingers, disrupting Miss Merk's lecture on the characteristics of Mars to announce, triumphantly, *"Kathryn burped!"*

I vow never to eat tuna burgers again.

To my right, a woman who wears a size six and is as skinny as those walking stick insects that resemble twigs, seems to be sucking in her waistline. Mine is the only abdomen in the class that protrudes more than two inches (it protrudes a good four inches, I'd say). I can't blame this bulge on children birthed thirteen or more years ago; surely I could have shed this baby weight sometime during the past decade.

But yoga should not be about comparing bellies. Surreptitiously, I glance at the gleaming diamond on the ring finger of the woman to my left, at the muscle in her thigh that bursts to life during our Warrior pose. Yoga isn't about gleaming diamonds, and I don't even care—for a moment—that my own engagement ring was a cheap opal that long ago cracked.

"This is not a competition," Ali scolds, glaring straight at me. As time passes, I will find that the yoga instructors have an uncanny talent for mind reading. Ali, with those deep, penetrating eyes, seems to see right through me. She is soft and hard at once; I sense sympathy and care as she watches me struggle, but I also sense impatience. I can tell that she'll have very little time for me if she ever hears me whine, "I can't" (my favorite mantra).

If it *were* a competition, clearly I would lose. As the other students chat in the hallway after class, I throw my mat into a cubby and hobble toward the door.

Outside, I stop and breathe in the night air, glancing up and down the avenue before crossing the street to the hill that winds to my house. Maybe this is a huge mistake, though it seems uncanny that a yoga center has cropped up just around my corner. I seriously wonder if I should go back again even though my therapist has prescribed it; if I do, I *must* buy some stylish yoga clothes. Like a clown, I've come to class in old purple sweatpants and a t-shirt; the others are all dressed in Lycra and high-fashion black!

Rock music blasts through our hallways, as if we live in a college dorm, but I'm making an attempt to get to sleep before midnight so that I'll be bright and chipper for tomorrow morning's yoga. I don't *want* to go, and yet I'm compelled to continue, if for no other reason, because I'd rather do yoga than take beta-blockers or Prozac. Well, not that the therapist has recommended Prozac, anyway, but she *has* suggested that it's not acceptable to waken in the night with palpitations and sweaty palms, envisioning crashing airplanes just because you're sending your son off to summer school in England (I'm not a psychic, after all). And it is not copasetic, she claims, to close one's eyes and see cars bounding up over curbs to flatten your children, or killer bees raining down from nowhere, or rabies being spread by neighborhood squirrels. Not on a regular basis, anyway.

Add these images up over fifty-some years, and you have a rather tense way of life. But that's how my mom lived, and it's how I live, too. Certainly, it's how I've lived ever since my first child was born twenty-two years ago. Not coincidentally, the last time I flew on an airplane was when I was pregnant with Aaron, my first baby. I distinctly remember the trip home from the West Coast, where my husband Mitch had been touring with his quintet. I'd flown out to tell him in person the wondrous news that I was pregnant, but on the way home, as I boarded the plane, my legs nearly crumpled, and as I sat gazing out the window as we soared through the sky, I felt a deep sense of foreboding. Yes, I was happy to be a mother, but I was also experiencing a scary kinship with my own mom's fears. For the first time in my life, I actually felt as if I really *was* my mother, as if I had truly accepted from her hands a symbolic mantle of motherhood that would keep me literally grounded for the next two decades (I'd never wear my mother's *real* clothes— she was partial to horrid little cotton housedresses that snapped up the front). Like my mother, I became terrified of traveling by air— with or without my children— and so, like my mother, I didn't do either from that day forth, as if, with motherhood, I'd morphed overnight from a relatively carefree career girl to a neurotic housewife in sloppy clothes.

Three years after that pivotal plane ride, Mitch arrived home from an opera rehearsal bursting with excitement. "We're going to China!" he cried. "Pack your bags!"

Aaron and I were busy on the floor, engaged in a marathon bout of Candyland. I gazed up at my husband and gathered Aaron tightly in my arms. Surely the man was delusional! "Uh…I don't think so. I couldn't possibly leave the baby, and I'm certainly not lugging him to the Far East."

"Come on, this is a great chance! Beverly Sills is letting spouses fly at a bargain rate! They're opening a brand new theatre in Taipei, and the opera's going to play at the inaugural performance! They're putting us up in the best hotels!"

"No way," I groaned, clutching Aaron to my chest.

"We can leave him with my parents?" Mitch asked hopefully.

"Not on your life. Besides, what if the plane crashes? Our baby will be an orphan! You'll just have to go without me."

For the next twenty years, whenever Mitch was called to fly to an exotic locale (or *any* locale), I stayed home, for the weight of the fear that kept me behind was far too heavy to lift.

And now, the fear has become outlandishly wide, threatening to spread its noxious arms into the lives of my children as they become young adults, just as my mother's fears spread into mine. Now, with my middle son heading across the Pond, my fear seems to be reaching a climax, and I can see that it's ever so close to stopping my sons from embracing their world. This is something that I can't allow. If I don't thwart this soon, I'll not only cause my boys to resent me, but I'll spend my golden years knitting in a rocking chair (perhaps without the knitting needles, which could be dangerous!) But make no mistake; this is not about blaming motherhood or blaming my beloved mother. It's about finding a way out.

Even my dear friend Anneke, who's very indulgent of my foibles (as I am of hers), has observed that my anxiety about my middle son's upcoming trip to England is over the top. In fact, it was Anneke who suggested I visit the therapist and gave me the name of a woman who helped her own mom when she suffered from a dash of agoraphobia. One day, after listening to me rant about Sam's chances of survival, Anneke pulled a piece of paper from her bag and wrote down a number.

"You need to see someone," she said.

"I'm sort of *afraid* of shrinks."

"You need to see someone *now*," Anneke insisted.

Since Anneke is a retired nurse (as well as my former next-door neighbor), I tend to take her medical suggestions to heart. After all, this wasn't the tone of voice she uses when she says, "I don't like this brand of Beaujolais" or "Toss me that pack of cigarettes." Visiting a shrink was an extreme measure for me—I'm not the sort of person who goes to doctors unless I'm running a high temperature (my mother often described herself as "a nervous wreck" yet she'd never even consider burdening a stranger with her problems). But under pressure from Anneke and with Mom gone, I reluctantly went for help, quivering nervously all the way to the therapist's office, where I followed a slim, kindly shrink into her inner sanctum, reluctant to reveal anything at all about myself.

"Tell me about your childhood," the therapist began, and within moments I was blubbering full force over my mother's death and my son's impending plane trip.

The therapist tossed me a Kleenex, her face oddly brightening, as if she suddenly remembered she had a secret key hidden away in her pocket.

"You could take beta-blockers," she began, "Or..."

"*Or?*"

"You could do yoga!"

"*Yoga?*"

It seemed like an odd suggestion, but since it didn't involve high speeds in a moving vehicle and was unlikely to cause a life-threatening allergic reaction (I've always been wary of pills as I'm sure I'd experience every side effect listed on a bottle), I wiped my eyes and sighed, "At least it's worth a try." (The thought of antidepressants and panic-reducing meds made me feel depressed and panicked.) Yoga ought to be harmless, I figured, unless I was intending to sleep on a bed of nails, which I most certainly wasn't.

I settle in under my covers, pulling the quilt over my ears. I can still hear wailing guitars and drumbeats, and now I also can make out the sounds of Mitch puttering in the kitchen a floor beneath our bedroom. It's his habit to nibble pretzels and have a cup of tea while watching Charlie Rose after a performance. Usually I sit with him and sip wine.

But not tonight.

∞

One week later, I'm here yet again at yoga. I wonder if Natalie, the cheerful woman who runs this yoga center, will consider me a stalker. Most of the participants come to one class a week. I'm attending twice or more, because I'm eager to learn and because I really do want to conquer the anxious beating of my heart, which has worsened since 9/11—a stupendous example of the Iceberg Theory if I ever saw one— and my mother's death two weeks before that.

I'm embarrassed by my ineptitude, but the only way to overcome it is by practice. Every Tuesday, I force myself to rise at eight o'clock, shower, eat a light breakfast of one hard-boiled egg and sip some tomato juice. Today, I creep away from the house, leaving my husband and sons sleeping. Sam, my fifteen-year-old, is flying to England in two weeks to study at Oxford for a month. (He's my over-achiever, the exact opposite of myself, and a perfectly adventuresome reflection of my husband Mitch, who never thinks of anything frightening unless it is actually happening.) I have imagined nothing but planes crashing and terrorist plots for the past forty eight hours. To be honest, I've thought of little else but planes crashing ever since Sam sent his application in to this program months ago. That and the doomed course that our country as a whole seems to be on. I feel the craziness of life on both a personal and national level.

Today I'm trying out a new teacher; I'm sure she'll be disgusted by my awkwardness. Yet as I enter the room, and see her sitting on her mat, I feel oddly reassured. She's blue-eyed and freckled, about five foot two. Her red hair is in tightly gelled ringlets, and she looks about thirty—twenty years younger than I. Peeking from her low-rider yoga pants is an awesome sunburst tattoo. As the seasoned mother of three children, I may have much more to teach this foxy young woman than she can teach *me*. But not about yoga.

"Hi! I'm Jill," she smiles grandly. "Have you practiced before?"

I nod my head. "A few times."

"Just do what you can."

I settle on my mat with a blanket and bolster. Supposedly, sitting on a blanket raises your "sit bones," and the bolster can be used for various "heart-opening" poses, some of which feel more, to me, like lounging on "the rack."

The class quietly fills with women who look to be in their thirties and early forties. Jill begins, "When you're worrying about something that may take place in the future, imagine the best thing that could happen, then think of the worst, then bring yourself to the middle—or most likely—scenario. Most of our fears are based on extreme scenarios, but that's not usually what happens." As I listen, tears roll down my cheeks. Is it possible, I marvel, that this woman somehow knows Sam is flying away?

I tiptoe up to Jill after class. "Thank you so much for the words of wisdom," I whisper.

She shakes her head, "It's the *yoga*—not *me*."

"Whatever it is, I appreciate it. I had no idea that yoga was anything like this."

Jill nods. "I had no idea when *I* started, either. But it changed my whole life."

"What did you do before?"

"I was a paralegal. When I discovered yoga, I left that world behind."

My eyes widen. I can't imagine this young woman in stockings and a suit. She looks like she was born in Lotus position, clad in baby-sized Spandex panties, toe rings and ankle bracelets.

Jill turns to another student, as if she's said enough. This teacher, I will come to learn, is a private person, more willing to share her touch and gaze than details about her life.

But that's okay with me! I don't really want her to know how screwed up *I* am, either.

∽

My sister is visiting for a few days from North Carolina, and it's a glorious late June weekend. Ruthann knows I'm hysterical about Sam leaving for England, so she offers to guide me through some kind of stress management technique that involves "tapping" gently on a number of the body's pressure points, while reciting a series of phrases (she's been a "New Ager" for ages). The whole thing sounds crazy, but that's my sister for you, even though tapping and chanting are just not things that we Livingstons do. At least they're not something my mother, father, brother or *I* do; Ruthann's always been a maverick, and for some reason she was able to shake off the doom and gloom that surrounded us as children. Perhaps it was because I was the youngest (my siblings are eleven and thirteen years older than I), or perhaps, like me, my parents became even more fearful as they aged, so I received the brunt of their neurosis. In any case, one of my clearest memories of my upstate New York childhood comes in the form of my mother's daily warning. Each and every time I would race out the back screen door, whether I was just going up to the corner mailbox or down the street to my best friend Beth's to play, I'd hear my mother's voice echo behind me.

"Be careful!" she would call. "*Be careful!*"

I wasn't even sure what I was supposed to be careful *of.*

So it seems that my past has become a bit of a problem, and I'm open to anything that might make that shapeless omnipresent fear recede. (My father—who held the reputable position of County Director of Probation— had his own phrasing for putting the hex on risk-taking. He'd simply say, "No. You can't *do* that.") But my dad's paranoia was not totally unfounded; his father had died out of the blue on New Year's Day in 1925 at the age of forty-six after confusing his heart meds, leaving his wife with four children and a farm. Within two years, the family watched their home go up in flames after it was bought by the railroad, which, in the name of progress and bigger trains, opted to alter the curve of the track so that it ran smack through my grandma's kitchen. As a child, I often heard such stories recounted time and time again; the tale of how my aunt contracted meningitis as a toddler and nearly died, the distant grandfather who went out to kill a deer for his family and was scalped by Indians.... And then, of course, my own dad's two heart attacks and stroke; I remember waking in the night, watching as he was carried away on a stretcher. There was clearly a sense that something terrible could happen at any moment, because in my family's history, it often *had.*

And if a personal tragedy weren't imminent, my parents would borrow from the woes of others, recounting accidents and illnesses culled from the newspaper or friends from church. After supper, they'd retire to the living room, where Dad would sit in an overstuffed chair and crackle his newspaper. "Did you read this piece about the poor kid who fell into French's Creek? Dead by the time they got to him."

Mom would shake her head and note, "Yes, and there's also a story about William Lane from up by Mariaville. He lost both his legs in that accident."

I'd sit on the floor at Dad's feet, reading the cartoons, and I couldn't help overhearing their commentary. They didn't seem to *want* to keep these grim tales secret, anyway, as if they thought by scaring the pants off me early on such a fate might be avoided. Though my parents never went out to dinner or to the movies, they attended many a wake and funeral; for a couple who rarely socialized, I always marveled at how many dead people they seemed to know.

Even minor illnesses were treated fearfully in my house. "*Pink eye!*" my mother would cry, holding my head between her hands. "It looks like *pink eye!*" The tone of her voice made me think that my eyes would be permanently discolored, or worse, that I might go blind. Or, "That's not impetigo, is it? *Not impetigo!*" a favorite affliction I never had and never would get. There was no such thing as a "leap of faith" in my house; it was all about a "leap of fear." A pain in the stomach automatically meant appendectomy (it didn't help that my sister actually needed one).

Over the years, my mother and I discussed the usual things like fire, tornados, wars, bombs, cancer, and AIDs. Then there were the racier items; drugs and drug dealers, aliens, terrorists, and the Bermuda Triangle. Choking on fish bones and ectopic pregnancies were biggies. Mom and I always dissected our fears together; now that I'm without her, I realize I don't really want to face them alone.

Perhaps then, the only way to handle this is to get rid of them, and if the therapist, yoga, and tapping are pathways to some kind of peace, what the hell. So I tag along as my sister leads me out to our deck underneath the apple blossoms in the warm spring air, and I follow as she chants and taps her fingers on her head and upper body, as if we're playing Simon Says.

"Now, you need to do this whenever you feel anxious," Ruthann explains. "You can tap gently wherever you are, without making a big show of it. As you tap, just repeat a phrase that describes your fear. Let's try 'fear of Sam getting on an airplane' for today."

My sister is now a hospice nurse (she changes occupations quite frequently, having been an elementary school teacher, psych nurse, stress reduction counselor, vegetarian restaurant waitress, chambermaid, and real estate agent in the past thirty years while I have remained one thing only— a writer). She is serene and smiling during this process, while I approach this ritualistic behavior with the same kind of mistrust and trepidation as I do my yoga class. But Ruthann, who is just over sixty, has always been easygoing, with the trusting, beatific face of a child. I remember being in tears at my sister's fiftieth birthday party—I was only thirty-nine at the time, and horrified that Ruthann was getting so old. My sis looked absolutely gorgeous in her flowing, India-print dress, and was given nifty incense, candles and "healing" crystals.

Out on the deck, I breathe in the scent from the enormous linden tree down the block. This same scent wafts up my hill every June, no matter what's going on in my life. So much seems to be in flux, but this heavy airborne perfume is the same every year at this time. I take comfort in things that remain the same. I like the fact that my apple tree blossoms every year, and I can expect the tulips to poke up in exactly the same spot next to my doorway each April. I don't like the fact that my mom is gone, that I'm getting older and that my little boys now need to shave. I'd prefer to be in a perpetual state of, say, age thirty-five. The world is moving far too fast for me, and if I can't slow it down, at least I need to find a way to stumble along.

I gaze up at my sister; her eyes are closed and she's swaying gently in the sunlight as she taps, her blondish-grey hair glistening. Secretly, I think my sister is totally out of her mind. And yet it is *she* who is calm and focused.

CHAPTER TWO: JULY

Breathe, Twist,
But Please Don't Shout

The sun is shining brightly this morning and I jettison from the bed like a rocket. This is it; the day Sam leaves for England, the day my fifteen-year-old baby boards an airplane all alone and flies into the great blue beyond without his mother. This is the day I must offer my middle son up to the gods; the day I must somehow live through without letting Sam suspect that I'm *sure* he's about to die.

I know plenty of people plunk their fifteen-year-olds on airplanes and let them fly overseas without batting an eyelash, but this is just not something we do in "my family," that is, in the family in which I grew up. My father (bless his wonderful soul) never even flew on an airplane in all of his eighty-one years; my parents never even once left the country. A trip to the Adirondacks in the summer was about as far as my parents ever went—and even that was rife with potential danger. As a teenager, I loved to paddle a kayak out to the middle of the lake where we vacationed, sit leisurely reading a Hemingway novel—I was heavily into Hemingway then and pleased to learn some years later that he had his own Iceberg Theory, which had to do with writing—hoping that a boy might pass by in a speedboat to stir up some waves. But my mother would always be on the shore with her binoculars, making sure that I didn't unzip my life preserver, frantically waving a white hankie over her head to summon me in if a thundercloud came near. No, my parents would definitely not approve of their grandson's excellent overseas adventure.

As Sam showers, I prepare a breakfast of eggs and juice, lightly buttering some toast. This excursion nearly caused him to miss my blackberry pie—an annual July tradition—but this year the bramble patch burst out a bit early and I was able to make one pie before Sam's departure. There's just one slice left in the frig, and I put that out on the table as well.

After Sam eats, we throw his backpack and suitcase into the car; Mitch is driving, and I hop into the passenger seat while Sam settles into the back. We don't talk much as we drive to the airport, other than my compulsory nagging: "Do you have your passport? Where is your cell phone? Where is that list of emergency numbers I gave you?" I'm a bundle of nerves, but Mitch believes a trip to England is just fabulous. He's more worried about how we're going to pay the exorbitant fee (just over $5000 for the month-long session), even though his mom and dear Anneke (who my kids think of as their aunt) have offered to pitch in. Money is the last thing on my mind; I'm just afraid my baby will fly into the horizon and never return.

Sam, who is nearly six feet tall, with beautiful lean muscles and an easy smile, is upbeat. We check his luggage, grab a last-minute bagel for him to munch on the plane, and head toward the gate. At the security check, Sam hugs me so tightly my ribs crackle;

then he lopes away with a last wave and grin, passing through the metal detector and disappearing into a vast, motherless universe.

As we lose sight of him, my tears erupt and my knees buckle. "He'll be spending his sixteenth birthday away from us!" I sob, as if I hadn't thought of this before.

Mitch grabs my arm, "Let's get you a drink." He guides me to a nearby airport bar and orders me a glass of wine while I sit shaking. Even though it's a trifle early in the day, I throw it back and ask for another. I guess all that "tapping" and yoga-ing hasn't really kicked in yet; alcohol sure seems like a speedier remedy. Still, I suppose the fact that I'm actually allowing Sam to do this is *something*. I know exactly what *my* parents would have said if I'd ever asked to go to Europe. "You can't *do* that!"

We meander around the airport until Sam's plane takes off. My son has never been so far away from me before, yet *I'm* the one who is weak in the knees and breathless. I think back to his first day of pre-school. With all my boys it was the same thing; I'd leave them whimpering in the classroom and I'd go home and cry for three hours. When I'd return, all red-faced and slobbery, they'd be happily playing with toy trucks. Sam in particular always made the transition to a new situation far faster than his mom. The pre-school teachers would always say the same thing: "He did great! Are *you* okay?"

Once Sam is up in the air, I think even Mitch feels a tad nervous, yet there's nothing we can do but wait. We stare at each other in weak disbelief and then head home. Somehow I get through the rest of the afternoon, but by evening I'm in panic mode again. Mitch whistles around the house before bed. "How about we snuggle up together and watch a movie?" he suggests.

"I don't think so, hon."

Instead, I sit up half the night with a bottle of chardonnay, "tapping" my damn brains out, finally stumbling to bed at daybreak. As I crawl under the covers, Mitch snorts in his sleep and rolls over. I want to shake him and scream, "There may be planes crashing in England! There may be terrorists on board!" But I force myself to close my eyes, and slowly drift away just as the first birds of morning begin to chatter.

At 6 a.m., the phone rings and I leap from the bed, grabbing for the receiver, knocking a slew of photos off my nightstand. Sam has arrived in England; the lofty educators who run the program have collected him, and he'll spend the next month in pure bliss, studying architecture, archaeology and anthropology, and threatening to visit a "hookah" lounge. The plane hasn't blown up and he hasn't been hijacked by terrorists. He hasn't been abducted by slave traders nor lost all his money and the pricey international cell phone I've rented. None of the horrors I've imagined have come to pass!

"Are you really okay?" I press.

"I'm fine, Mom! *Chill*. At ease!"

My mother let me drink from her cup of panic. I just hope I can keep my poison to myself.

We're deep into the sweltering days of July, and I've been at yoga now for ten sessions. When my alarm rings at eight, I imagine turning it off and going back to sleep. I am too old for yoga. My muscles still tremble from Tuesday's session, and I know I won't be able to hold that damn Downward Dog pose while Ali croons, "take five deep breaths," the longest deep breaths I've ever inhaled. Yes, I am way too old for yoga, though I know that's just an excuse since my seventy-five-year-old mother-in-law can dive into the Dolphin pose like an Olympic swimmer. (She's the mirror of my husband and the two share such an aggravating "can do" attitude toward life.) But age, really, has nothing to do with yoga. "We are all beginners," said Ali solemnly at the end of my last session.

I roll over and snap off the alarm before it can disrupt all the sleeping male forms in my home. Sam is still in England, and Ben, my thirteen-year-old, Aaron, who is home from college for three months, and Mitch, who works till midnight, will gladly sleep for hours yet. I pull my new, regrettably form-fitting yoga pants from the drawer and head to the shower. I nibble a hard-boiled egg and drink a quarter-inch of juice. No coffee. No one, I've observed, ever leaves Jill's class to pee, as if in a moment of absence, one might miss some earth-shattering, yogic revelation.

At nine, I stroll down to the Yoga Center and enter the studio, surprised to find that the teacher subbing for Jill today is a lanky male with a quiet, humorless manner. He has the long hairy legs of Kafka's Gregor and a reedy voice. His eyes are the color of a dark, hot swamp.

As we move through the poses, my mind shifts. I no longer feel old. I am weak, I tremble, yet I hold the Warrior pose, I manage a Plank pose, I lower to Cobra, and then rise to the damn Downward Dog. In Triangle, we shift our weight to the left and then stretch the right arm as far as it will go before tipping over, the left arm raised up to the ceiling. As I balance, my mind seems to clear.

At the end of the session, our "Om" is oddly lacking harmony, with the teacher's voice an octave below the searching voices of the eight women who join him. Yet when I open my eyes, I don't even know how old I am. I've totally forgotten that I am the oldest person in the room. In fact, I've forgotten that I'm even *in* this room, as if I've miraculously left my body. Wouldn't *that* be grand!

∽

A warm July rain falls in torrents before class tonight, but I drive to the center. I'd like to just chuck this venture overboard, but I've made a commitment. I have to give this a few months at least, to see if it helps me feel any less anxious. The fact that I'm anxious about *going* to yoga, however, is worrisome. And I admit that I've never been a joiner. I've always been turned off by pack mentality, and mindless, grinning, guru-followers incessantly nibbling on seeds and nuts. Still, I'd rather twist my body around than habitually pop pills.

Tonight, two new students show up; one is older than I. Tonight, *I'm* the "experienced" one, and the session is easier than usual. I'm relieved, yet find myself almost wishing for the pain that comes from trying to keep up with the tight-bellied younger women who've been doing yoga for ten years, the women I privately think of as the "power yoginis." (A yogini, I've learned, is a female who practices yoga; a yogi is male. Who knew?)

Tanya, the svelte Asian instructor who leads this evening class, reminds us to breathe slowly. "The yogis," she reveals, "believed that we are each born with about five billion breaths. The longer our breaths, the longer will be our lives."

I wonder if that's just wishful thinking on the yogis' part. It could be that people who take longer breaths just don't get as many breaths into their lifespan. But I tend to think negatively, and apparently the yogi mentality requires a more positive outlook. I realize that at the end of a session, I never feel breathless. I feel breath-full.

The breath is a curious thing. When I was a child, I often felt as if I had lost my breath completely, and I remember nights of tears and panic as I fought to regain it. My parents insisted my breathing problems were caused by dust (though Mom was forever dusting) or animal hair (Princess Bonnie Lassie, our snarling cocker spaniel who hung out under our back porch, was not exactly a glamour queen). For years in early childhood—but only at bedtime when I lay alone in the dark—I felt as if my breath came in and seemed to get stuck in my throat. Then I'd cry until Mom snuggled next to me or Dad gently caressed my forehead. My fear literally took my breath away, but I don't know why or where it went.

When I arrive home from Tanya's class, Mitch is lounging on the deck sipping a cup of cappuccino before he takes off to play a late-program piece at the New York City Ballet. It unnerves me to see him still here when he has a minimum one hour door-to-door commute to Lincoln Center *without* traffic, but he's used to slipping into the pit at the last second, and nothing, short of moisture in his clarinet pads (which causes horrifying squawks), rattles Mitch.

My husband sets his coffee mug down on the railing. "Are you learning anything?" he demands.

"I'm learning *something* all right. I just don't know *what.* "

"I certainly hope so," he observes. He's a pragmatic sort who doesn't approve of luxuries like hot tubs, pedicures or cable TV. Mitch's idea of a walk is a *five-mile* walk, and I know he won't support the idea of yoga just for "fun."

"I hope this isn't Romper Room yoga," he sneers as he exits. "I want to see some *results.*"

The "power yoginis"—a group of about six women, all friends, all proficient, all attired in the latest yoga fashions with perfectly polished nails—are here again and the class is full on this sunny morning. As I sit in Sukhasana (cross-legged position), I fight the urge to flee. I've heard of a woman who did that; she crept out the door while everyone's eyes were closed because she was so afraid she'd make a fool of herself. I know this feeling all too well, this feeling of not belonging, of being unable to fit in or keep up. It's not just about yoga, this feeling that's dogged my life; it's also about working, being a mom, being a wife, doing just about everything I do.

I suppose it's no mystery where this comes from. My mother

gave up college to get married after one year and never pursued her dream to be a teacher; her whole life, she alluded to her lack of education, although she was as bright as anyone I've ever known, and she read relentlessly. My mom always felt that she didn't measure up; her rambling Victorian was outdated and dilapidated compared to the women from town who lived in brand new ranch houses, and her clothes were from JC Penny's, not Lord and Taylor. She felt just terrible that she'd never finished college; she doubted herself, and so I doubted myself, too.

Mom was a professional fretter, and if *I* was worried that my father might die before his time, you could be sure that my mother was haunted by the possibility, not only because she loved him but because she literally didn't know what she'd do without him. She had no college degree, no work experience and a nervous constitution—my dad was always racing to get Mom's smelling salts out of her handbag when she'd begin to "swoon." She'd married the man at the age of seventeen—he was thirteen years her senior and her former high school teacher— and fell swiftly into the role of homemaker. Mom hung on Dad's every word, though she never literally hung on *him*—public displays of affection were uncommon in my family, except between mother and child. But Dad was her rock, and she adored him; they made a handsome couple, too, for my father was a professorial-looking guy with wire-rimmed glasses who folks always described as "a gentleman," and my mom, though "pleasantly plump," had the innocent beauty of an Ingrid Bergman (she was quite slim when she married I found out when I once tried to squeeze into her navy blue wedding outfit).

Today my muscles tremble with fatigue, as if my body has been sleeping for at least thirty years. I'm Rip Van Winkle in stylish gray stretch capris! I try to hold the Triangle pose, but my legs are near to collapsing. When we move to the Downward-Facing Dog—the "resting pose," as the instructor calls it in a tone I personally interpret as sarcasm—I fall softly into Child's pose. Tanya places her hand on my shoulder and whispers, "Do only as much as you can."

During Savasana—the minutes at the end of each class truly devoted to resting, with our legs splayed and our arms at our sides in Corpse pose—Tanya hesitates at each mat. I can hear her tiptoeing near, but I don't dare open my eyes. We're like children pretending to be asleep in our beds. Tanya comes closer, then reaches and gently squeezes the soles of my feet. I smile softly, for I've forgotten, once again, both how old I am, and how much I wanted to leave.

Even so, I'm still uncomfortable. Yoga feels a bit like a foreign country, and I don't travel well. And yet I'm less uncomfortable here than I was the last time I stepped into a traditional church (I was raised Presbyterian, or as my husband says, *repressed*byterian). There's something calming about this place, and I'm beginning to sense that people come to yoga again and again the way they might climb to the same spot on a hilltop or to a familiar rock by a gentle stream. Is it just dumb luck or something grander that has planted a yoga center on my street?

Oh happy day! It's July 31 and Sam returns this morning from England. We drive to the airport, laughing and chatting all the way. Though terrorists and crashes are still on my mind, they don't seem as imminent on the return trip. We park the car and race to the gate where Sam will soon miraculously materialize.

When he strides into view, Mitch and I wave frantically; I grab the first hug. We gather his bags and head for the car, pulling onto the New Jersey Turnpike. Sam chatters about his trip, but his eyes soon glaze over and he tires of my questions: "Did you make a lot of friends? Were your teachers nice? You didn't really go to that Hookah lounge?"

"Chill," Sam commands. He needs to sleep for a day or so.

We pull into our driveway in less than half an hour and unload Sam's few bags. I've planned a welcome home lunch, but our son says he's too exhausted to eat and heads to his bedroom. Even with his door closed and his pile of bags and dirty laundry in the hallway, it feels wonderful to have him home. I'm so much happier when all my sons are here. My mom was this way too; I learned how to "let go" from my mother, which basically means it's a lesson we never covered. We got to the PhD level, however, in our studies of holding on for dear life.

Fear and doubt held hands like dance partners in my family, and Mitch spent the first few years of our marriage trying to pry them apart. I'd been waltzing with my doomsayer shadow since childhood, and he had to cut in and say, "Let *me* take over here!" Before we were married, Mitch lived in a rat and roach-infested apartment on Manhattan's upper West Side with two other music students. As we climbed into Mitch's loft to make love, I often heard a French horn honking on the other side of the paper-thin wall; simultaneously, the other roommate, a gangly Kansas City boy, would be squeaking his oboe reeds—a shrill, turkey-murdering kind of sound. Prior to its gentrification, this area of New York was quite colorful; we had to weed through bums swilling whiskey on the building's front steps and often we passed transvestites in the stairwell, dressed for an evening on the town. Obviously, my parents had no clue I was staying with Mitch here; I told them that when I visited from college, or later from my newspaper job in New Paltz, New York, I was bunking at Mitch's wealthy uncle's lovely brownstone in an upscale neighborhood. Having been raised and educated in upstate New York, and having started my career in the Hudson Valley, my first trips to Mitch's bachelor pad were terrifying, but I was smitten with a classical clarinetist and there was no turning back.

Sure, there had been other guys in high school and college who pursued me (and a few whom I had pursued), but I was drawn back to Mitch like a magnet every time I strayed. I don't know what it was exactly that drew us together, other than the basics like great sex and similar politics, but there was definitely something more. I always felt "right" when I was with Mitch, and once in a while, when I envisioned marrying someone else, I felt the kind of nauseating dip in my stomach I'd get on a Ferris wheel, the kind that made me scream, "Get me off of this thing *right now!*" Once, when Mitch and I were kissing under the stars in a field near our hometown, I felt something strange, as if we were getting the "nod" from a higher location. It wasn't that the earth moved...but I definitely felt that the spray of Northern Lights above us was reflecting what was going on in our hearts. He was a bit of an odd dude (most of the guys I dated at least drank beer now and then, and Mitch was the only one I'd ever met who could spend an entire evening discussing Vivaldi or Charles Ives), but there was no getting around the fact that I was in love with him. It didn't hurt that he was so totally "out there" with his feelings for me, either. I'd never met a guy before who brought up the subject of marriage on the third date, or who would stare so deeply and endlessly into my eyes.

When we tied the knot in 1977, Mitch found a slightly better building in Washington Heights, but after living in New Paltz, with its gentle streams and stupendous mountain views, our fifth floor walk-up was a downer. Mitch was excited to show me our first apartment: a small, dreary living room, a tiny kitchen with six different patterns of contact paper stuck to the walls, a miniscule bath with a rusty tub, and a narrow, slanted bedroom. I glanced out the window at the brick building view, sank down on my knees, and cried my heart out. How could I ever call this home?

But there was one good thing about the apartment. When I phoned my childhood friend Beth to tell her I'd be moving to Manhattan, she was thrilled, since she'd just started nursing school there. "What's your address?" she asked.

"Umm…. let's see here. West One Hundred and Seventy… I think it's between Broadway and Fort Washington Avenue."

"That's not possible!" Beth laughed. "*I* live on West One Hundred and Seventieth Street on the corner of Fort Washington."

"Are you *sure?*"

"Of course I'm sure! I moved in here two months ago. I *told* you my new place was in upper Manhattan!"

In all of the City's apartments, Mitch had chosen ours based on the affordable rent without even knowing that Beth lived just up the block. My whole life was changing, but the friend who had lived around the corner when I was five to eighteen years old was still just around the corner, and that was a blessing.

It was here that I learned what it was really like to be married to a struggling classical musician—sort of like being wed to a doctor who was always on call, except that the money wasn't in it. Mitch's favorite place to perform in the early years of our marriage was 56th Street and Fifth Avenue. That's right, on the street, where he and his quintet members would play their own arrangements of popular and classical works. On a good night Mitch would come home with $40 in his pocket, but more often 20 bucks or less for three or four hours of work. The basic mix was two women (the flute and bassoon) and three men (clarinet, French horn and oboe). Their original name was The Caloroso Quintet, derived from the Italian *calore*—warm and passionate. But after an Hispanic onlooker called out, "Hey man! In Spanish your name means hot and sweaty!" they changed it to The Linden Quintet. Of course, on those steamy nights in the dead of summer, hot and sweaty was precisely what they were.

During the first year of our marriage, I worked as a writer and editor at a trade magazine until the company moved out of state and an old college friend called to offer me a job at a photography magazine where she was an editorial assistant. With much trepidation, I agreed.

When I reported for duty I discovered that Trina, the friend who had promised to walk me through my first week, was out with a broken arm. So I'd have to handle this new job on my own for a while, including dealing with the savvy, caustic, cosmopolitan staff. On my first day, the managing editor—an efficient young woman in a suit and heels— greeted me with a toppling stack of photographs to be returned to their rightful owners.

"I'd like you to *very* carefully slip each image between two sheets of cardboard, and then place the cardboard into an envelope. Whatever you do, make sure the photograph is well protected!" she instructed. "Here's my Rolodex; it has everything you need."

"Sure!" I smiled. "Piece of cake," I thought to myself, though the pile itself was daunting.

I started sifting through, stopping after a few easy returns. "Um, I don't see an address for Roger Fenton on your Rolodex," I chided. "Can you tell me where I can find him?"

My new boss rolled her eyes. "That would be difficult. No doubt he's moved around a bit since his death in 1869."

I had much to learn, but I stuck with it, working my way up the masthead. Of course, I volunteered only to write articles about dead photographers who could be researched in library books or those who lived in New York City and its environs, while Trina flew off to Kenya and Australia, and the others visited the Middle East, Europe, and the West Coast on assignment. Even so, my job was exciting and challenging. I got to follow Ronald Reagan's personal photographer around the White House for a profile I was assigned to write, and I'd often go out for drinks with fashion photographers or photojournalists. I sat sipping French Lillet with the famed Andre Kertesz in his apartment not long before he died, and I was always running to openings and book signings where models, photographers and editors gathered, some dressed to the nines.

My husband's world was music and mine was words. I left our apartment before Mitch got up in the morning and went to bed before he rolled in at midnight or later. My life was the photography magazine and my friends there; they turned out to be a hilarious, fun-loving bunch I grew to adore. Mitch, meanwhile, was trying to establish his career, and in the process we often clashed. He began to suspect, quite rightly, that I seemed more married to the magazine than I did to him. But he was not a young man who would sit down to discuss a problem; in those days, he'd simply shut off his emotions, and stalk out the door.

Weirdly enough, this troubled time in our marriage came just at the point when my hormones had begun to whine for a baby, and it occurred to me that if I didn't have a baby with Mitch, it would be quite a chore to track down another man of his high caliber, develop a relationship strong enough to be parents, and set everything in motion. So even though we weren't getting along all that well, I broached the subject.

"Are you crazy?" he asked the first time I brought it up.

"Maybe. But I think I'd like to be a mother."

"I'd like to practice *more*, not less," Mitch would say.

"But doesn't it seem *natural* for two married people to have a baby?" Natural was a good argument with Mitch. He hated it when I wore lipstick or nail polish, and God forbid I should ever use chemical dye on my hair.

"Hmmm. I guess."

Finally, he agreed that he would give *one* baby a try. Mitch has always been a strong proponent of biological needs (especially his own), and, to his credit, he also realized that arguing against a woman's biological clock would be insanely futile.

Not long after we began thinking about having our first child, Mitch took off for the West Coast on a five-week tour with his quintet, and I seized the opportunity to work longer hours and party with friends. Two weeks into Mitch's trip, I was at a bar with Trina on a Friday after work, sipping a glass of wine, when I realized I felt queasy. Could I possibly be pregnant? I pushed the glass away and went home.

The next day, I bought a pregnancy test. Indeed, I was carrying a baby! In a frenzy, I decided to meet Mitch in Vegas, and I hopped on a plane. (Question: When does life begin? Answer: not until I'm too nervous to board an airplane!) As soon as we were alone that night I confessed all: not only was I pregnant, but also I'd been drinking a little more heavily than usual. I knew it wouldn't be fair to lie to Mitch, in case he didn't think we should go through with this pregnancy because of my carelessness.

Much to my surprise, Mitch threw his arms around me and jumped up and down! "This is wonderful news!" he cried.

"But...what about the wine?"

"That *was* stupid. But you're probably over-reacting. It's not as if you've been swilling bottles of booze for nine whole months."

"In those early weeks when the fetus is first forming, it's so vulnerable," I moaned.

"We can, and we *will* do this, no matter what." He held me close and I snuggled into his neck. At last, I felt like we would really be together in this.

"But what if there's something wrong with the baby?"

"Whatever life serves us we'll handle."

I was grateful that this was his attitude, because in my heart I agreed. I wanted that baby more than I'd ever wanted anything.

But though I didn't know it then, that baby would totally change the path of my career. Before long, I'd be interviewing Mr. Rogers instead of Patrick Demarchelier, and writing about colic, diaper rash and tantrums instead of fashion shoots or nudes.

Days of Wine and Whining

I'm shocked that I've been at yoga for two months; I was quite sure I'd have given it up by now, like that potato diet I tried a few years ago or my two-day attempt at jogging. But this seems different somehow. After all, my goal isn't just to lose some belly fat; it's also to trim the excess worry and heavy thoughts from my head.

Tonight Tanya says we should "find our mountain." She's talking about positioning our feet so that we feel balanced in Mountain pose. I realize that even with our feet firmly planted on our mats in Tadasana, we are each in our own way climbing our own mountain.

I've never really felt firm and tall on my own two feet, but now I begin to imagine what it might be like. I'm pleased with the feeling, with my eyes closed, of knowing I am holding myself up tall. I am not holding my parents' hands, or my husband's, and I'm not holding the hand of one of my children. I'm on my own in a dark, quiet room, and yet I feel as if I'm standing in a larger world. I'm alone in my thoughts, and I feel secure, yet I'm still afraid of where my thoughts might travel.

I'm not thinking of my age or the state of my body tonight. During Savasana, I secretly open my eyes and gaze toward the window. The sky is darkening, and I realize that the summer days are already becoming shorter. I imagine what it will be like to be here in this room in the wintertime, when snow is softly falling outside and the night is dark. This is a good sign, because it means I'm considering staying with yoga a bit longer.

With Sam back from England, my reason for going to yoga in the first place—to deal with my anxiety about his trip—is gone. Now I know that I have many more reasons for continuing, both physical and spiritual. "Sam will bring the world to you," as Anneke once said. "Maybe," she added, "you will one day want to step into that world yourself."

I met Anneke twenty years ago over our backyard hedge. She was my next-door neighbor first, and then my close friend, even after she moved to another street in our funky little mile-square town. Anneke, a tall woman with a thunderous laugh, has been all over the world and then some, and is now on her third husband. I've been with the same man for twenty-seven years and in the same house for twenty. I remember once telling Anneke that I'd already done everything I wanted to do, but she didn't believe me. "Don't you want to swim with dolphins or ride an elephant? Don't you want to glide down the Amazon River in a skinny canoe?"

"I might like to drink a good bottle of red wine in Paris," I admitted.

I've always feared the unfamiliar, but yoga is making me feel more open to possibilities. I can't understand why moving my body is helping to release my mind, yet this seems to be happening. I wonder if my fears will recede, whether I'll one day yearn to swim with dolphins, as Anneke does, or if a day will come when I won't be afraid to be alone with my own thoughts. I press my feet into my mat, my hands folded together at my heart. Somehow the simple act of standing tall makes me realize just how much metaphorical slumping I do.

In the morning, I meet with my therapist, and we mutually agree that I can stop coming. Sam is back from his trip, and my own journey has begun.

"I'll be happy to see you again if you feel the need," she offers, "but I think you're going to solve your problems. I can tell you're on your way because your mind is open."

I've reported that I've been dutifully going to yoga and I think she's impressed. She is a great advertisement for yoga; she's a yogini herself, with a gracious demeanor and a phenomenal body!

∞

The wiry male instructor is here again. This time, he starts with those dreadful breathing exercises: "Breathe through the top of your nostrils." This means absolutely nothing to me, but pranayama—a variety of breathing techniques—is a vital part of yoga. Every time an instructor explains one of these methods, I fake it like a woman who can't have orgasms. I fake sending my breath to my back, sending my breath to my belly, sending my breath anywhere. My breath just goes wherever the hell it wants to go. "Soften the belly," this guy instructs. Excuse me, sir, but my belly is soft enough!

He's in a good mood today, but he doesn't touch me, or any of the women. The female instructors press against our hips, massage our feet and necks, firmly push our legs wider, towering above us like Amazon warriors with yoga straps. Perhaps this is why I don't care for this dude; he hasn't touched me.

In Savasana, with my eyes closed and my body in Corpse position, the CD player slips into Bach's Air on the G String. I see a series of images: Mitch when we were first married, playing his clarinet with his open case on the streets of Manhattan; the walk home from the hospital with our first beautiful baby; our wedding day and the manner in which my father touched my elbow so tenderly as he guided me; my mother…no, I can't and won't see my mother, because it's still too painful to admit that she's gone. Tears slide from my closed eyes, and I fear, for a moment, that I'm about to die. I can think of no other reason to see these scenes from my life flashing before me. Is it already too late to rescue myself?

We roll to the fetal position, then to cross-legged sitting, our hands in prayer position or Anjali Mudra, pressed to our hearts. As I wipe my tears away with the palms of my hands, I realize that, somehow, I *have* been touched by this yogi.

Next week, Jill will be back.

Tanya says that Downward-Facing Dog is an "active pose." I could have *sworn* she told us before that it was a "resting" pose, and now I wonder if I got the whole thing wrong. When I leave class tonight, I feel bereft. Summer is waning, and since I'll be away next week, I won't see Tanya again for a while. I suppose this is the way people feel about their therapists, pastors or hairdressers. We become intimately attached to these people who are trying to help us (whether by calming our minds, our spirits, or our frizz). I wonder if I could center my entire life on yoga (people do, I've learned). I'm reminded of the way I felt with newborn babies; I was so devoted to my babies that I felt as if I lived and breathed only when they were in my arms. Yoga is sort of like this—I must be in the falling in love phase.

After a slapdash spaghetti dinner with the boys, I begin to clean up the kitchen, mentioning once again to Mitch that we really need a new dishwasher.

"We can struggle along with this," Mitch says, slamming shut the door of the appliance and positioning a chair against it so that the water won't spill out when we press "on."

"We really need a new one. Every morning there's a puddle on the floor, as if we have a puppy."

"We just don't have the money right now!"

Once Mitch leaves for work, I sit at my computer and surf some job sites. I've been considering getting a "real" job for a while and this dishwasher dispute has clinched it. I cruise around the job sites until I come across a position that seems promising; a writer's service agency is looking for someone to proofread. I click on my resume and position it as an attachment. But before I press "send," I jot a little note, explaining that I can only work three days a week, even though it's a fulltime position. No matter what, I need to preserve some time for writing— and for yoga.

Deep down, I know this effort is doomed; you don't get a job by telling the employer when you *can't* work. But I'd rather live a spiritually and physically healthier life than get a new dishwasher anyway, and because I have a husband who supports our family I can make this choice. Yes, our finances are hurting, but my time is more important than whatever I could buy if I didn't have it.

This is a lesson I began to learn when our first baby was born; becoming a mother makes you realize how truly little time there is in a given day. I took the customary three-month maternity leave from the magazine, and then returned to my office, designating Mitch as Aaron's daytime caregiver. The arrangement of a musician/stay-at-home dad seemed ideal, at first, but there were also a number of problems, not the least of which was the fact that Mitch could be called at the last minute to fill in for an established clarinet player who couldn't make a rehearsal, and if he wasn't available, future calls from that contractor would be forfeited. (The arts can be a cutthroat business; after all, there are only two or three clarinets in an orchestra, only a handful of orchestras in New York with a season long enough to offer a decent living, and hundreds of students studying to be clarinetists, not only at Juilliard and Manhattan School of Music, but in music departments all across the nation.) So he needed to line up some baby backups: a bassoonist who played in his quintet and a couple of attractive young Puerto Rican ladies from our apartment building in Washington Heights. While I was at my desk in midtown Manhattan or hobnobbing with fashion photographers and editors, my baby was home with a revolving door of sitters. Not exactly a healthy way to form a bonding attachment with a primary caregiver.

But as it turns out, the baby did fine. *I* was the *real* basket case. In my office, I'd sit staring at Aaron's picture on my wall, milk leaking from my breasts, tears dripping from my eyes, worrying about what might be going on at our apartment. I trusted Mitch with our baby—but the other caregivers had me worried sick.

One day, when Mitch was called to a last minute rehearsal and I was on deadline at the office, he begged his former roommate—a bachelor and French horn player—to pinch-hit for him. The guy had no experience with babies, but he was a kind soul.

As Mitch hurriedly gathered up his instruments, he gave his pal some last minute instructions. "The baby's sleeping now, but he might be cranky when he wakes up because he's teething. If he seems grouchy, just give him a biscuit!" Mitch suggested, tossing a box to his friend.

Hours later, I returned home from work to find Aaron standing in his crib in his diaper, wearing a silly grin, as if he knew— even at the age of ten months— that Mommy was not going to be happy he'd been given the green light to OD on

Zwieback. A dozen half-nibbled biscuits surrounded him on the mattress; biscuit bits dangled from the crib bumpers and hung from the creases in his diaper. In the corner of the crib was the biscuit box itself, flattened by Aaron's cute little feet.

"Thanks," I smiled wanly at the sitter as I led him to the door. I figured there wasn't much point in a lecture.

Once he was gone, I scooped my crumby little boy into my arms without taking off my work clothes, hugged him close and decided this couldn't go on. What kind of mother was I anyway?

If I wanted to be truly married to Mitch, someone's schedule would have to change because we couldn't keep up this parenting relay race, handing our baby back and forth like a baton and living separate lives. I worked throughout Aaron's first year, until I had enough saved to get a mortgage on a tiny house in New Jersey (Mitch didn't even qualify for a credit card), and then I quit. Our plan was for me to freelance, writing photography books and magazine articles. Mitch's career was beginning to take off. He was subbing more and more at the opera and had landed positions at the New York Chamber Symphony and several other small orchestras and bands. Together, we decided that we'd live modestly and make do. Our main goals were to raise our own children, write, and play music. We'd never be rich, but we'd be able to say that we had "followed our bliss." Besides, the seedling notion of a second baby had already implanted in my mind. A year after Aaron's birth, we followed our bliss to the suburbs.

Aaron was four when Sam arrived, and three years later, Ben was born. We'd decided that since I seemed to be getting along working at home, what was one more, or heck, two more babies? We wanted Aaron to have a sibling, but more than that, I just loved being a mother, and in spite of his early protests, Mitch was perfectly cut out for being a dad. When we first married, the idea of three children would have seemed absurd. But once we were in the thick of it, three was just the ticket. Besides, in spite of our complaining about how stressful parenting was and how much we needed more sleep, the bottom line was that we loved the little devils. They were naughty and wild, but at the end of the day, nothing gave me more pleasure than nursing my baby to sleep or reading the boys a favorite story. I was never much attracted to kids in the past—I was not one of those little girls who endlessly cooed over baby-dolls or dreamed of being a mommy—but once I had my own, my outlook on children flip-flopped. Oddly, though, it was Mitch who suggested we try for a trio.

"But I'd like to do *more* writing, not less!" I answered with surprise. Still, after I thought about it for a while, I realized that one more baby—boy *or* girl—*would* be perfect.

The silly thing was, I wanted it all—and I wanted it all without a nanny. Maybe I'd bitten off more than I could chew. I had three little boys, two magazine columns, a house that needed to be cleaned, a family that needed to be fed, and a host of other writing and mom-related duties. As they grew older, just coordinating their social and extracurricular activities was a full time occupation. The job was stressful and demanding, yet as most parents will avow, there's an uncanny reservoir of stamina and strength that arises when you're raising a child. You may not *think* you can make it up the steps chasing a toddler and carrying a baby and two bags of groceries, but you *do*. You may even do it with a smile on your face while singing "Itsy Bitsy Spider."

Mitch helped of course, but the juggling was frustrating, and Mitch was unreliable, his schedule prone to change at a moment's notice. And in some ways, my career was just as unpredictable as my husband's— I'd go for two months without an assignment and then three would come in at once. I felt like an insanely spinning top—was I a mommy at home with a baby, or —as I once saw myself described online—"a photo historian?" Well, certainly I was no historian! But I had a reputation as a reliable writer, and motherhood seemed to threaten that. Whenever I gave my attention to my work, something would go wrong with the family and whenever I focused on the family, something would go wrong with my work.

Those years of raising three rowdy boys were marvelous but rough, especially when they were younger. Yet sometimes, when Mitch would come riding home from Manhattan on his moped in his tuxedo with a bag of Chinese food slung onto his pack, I'd be overcome by gratitude. I felt very lucky to have married a man who cared enough about spending time with his children to race to New Jersey after his matinee, and then head back into the city after one hour home for dinner to play Figaro or Butterfly, for by then he had landed a half-year position at the opera (which runs just six months a year). But it wasn't all roses; plenty of days I wished I could just get the hell out of Jersey, motherhood *and* marriage itself.

"How was your afternoon?" Mitch would ask, idling his moped and tossing me the bag of takeout provisions—chicken low mien and wonton soup.

"Like demons have been eating at my brains."

Half the time, I didn't even know where to begin: the 40 gruesome cicada bug carcasses the boys had stuck on the screen door (of course, I'm terrified of insects; even more so of their ugly abandoned shells), the football they shot through the living room window, the hole kicked into the upstairs wall, the fact that they'd locked me out of my own house? Boys are boisterous, that's the bottom line, and even with the occasional high school babysitter called in for relief, I had my hands full.

"It can't be so bad," Mitch insisted.

He had no idea.

It's yoga morning again. On the way down my hill, I puzzle

over the money issue. Why am I spending money on yoga? To still my mind. But why is my mind rumbling about spending money on yoga? Because it's not yet still. This sounds like the kind of eternal paradox that the Buddha or some other spiritual master might be able to solve, but it sure isn't being solved by me.

I enter the Yoga Center and pull my mat from my cubby like a preschooler (unlike a rambunctious toddler, however, I tiptoe quietly into the room). Jill sits silently on her mat at the head of the class. Today, she begins with a story about the meaning of happiness.

"What really makes you happy?" she asks. "If it's your jewelry, then fine, enjoy it. But is it something else? Something you can't touch?"

I realize that it wasn't so crazy to send in a job application stipulating that I need two days off for writing and Jill's class each week. Anyway, I wonder how many of my life choices have been more about *fleeing* my fears than about *pursuing* happiness or anything else. At least I didn't wimp out when it came to motherhood.

We dig into our sun salutations and other asanas (pronounced *ahhh*-sa-nas, because of the ahhh you feel when you get them right?), trying to keep pace with our enthusiastic teacher. At the end of our session Jill leads us in three reps of "Om." All women, our voices match hers. One of us, however, is completely off key. She must be tonedeaf, yet her voice rings out loudly, her "Om" coarse and guttural. My eyes are closed, but it *seems* as if this awkward Om is coming from the most proficient of the yoga students in this class. Here's something I can do that she can't!

I give Jill a swift hug before I leave class, and she hugs me back, a serene little smile on her face. Maybe she's a bit surprised—but on the other hand, she sees me here every week, and she must suspect that this is really important to me.

I'll be away next week on vacation and I'll miss both Ali's and

Jill's classes. I hope that my practice doesn't regress—just when I'm beginning to make some progress. But obviously, I have a long way to go before I'm in a true yoga state of mind. If I were an authentic yogini, I certainly wouldn't be comparing the quality of our Om's as if we're woodwind players in an orchestra!

We have an entire week for vacation in the middle of August—a rare commodity for a musician who hates to turn down work. But now that Mitch is an established professional, we can risk leaving town.

We make the trip to the Cape in six hours; with my husband and boys, I'm visiting my dear friend Eloise, whom I met more than thirty years ago at Kirkland College in Clinton, New York. I feel comforted just being around Eloise and her family at their summer home; she's the kind of woman who tells *everyone* to button up their raincoat or help themselves to another cookie.

Eloise is my kindred spirit and yet we're totally different. She's a teacher of learning disabled high school kids, and though she's had tragedy in her life—she lost both of her parents to cancer a few years back—-she always wears a hopeful expression. At Kirkland, she was my suite mate, and over time, she's proven to be my true soul mate, in a way a husband can never be. When we first met (two girls on financial aid at a college where many in our dorm hailed from Park Avenue) we felt an immediate connection. There was something funny, quirky, and brilliant about this girl with thick, jet-black hair and an impish smile. I recall the first time she invited me into her room just across the hall.

"Sit down, but watch the rat!" she ordered.

I noticed a flash of white scurrying across her bedspread.

"Pilfered from the psych lab for the weekend," Eloise explained. "I've grown attached to the little guy. His name's Eugene."

We bonded so deeply and immediately that we've always

believed we were just "meant for each other."

So I'm thrilled to be spending a week with Eloise, but I also feel almost a sense of panic about getting to a yoga session. I'm afraid that if I miss my yoga classes I'll lose all that I've gained so far, and I don't want to jeopardize the flicker of peace I've been feeling lately.

As if she's been reading my thoughts, Eloise pulls me over to her computer after dinner. "Look what I found!" she smiles mischievously.

I bend over the screen to discover a yoga website advertising beach yoga at 7 a.m. tomorrow morning. "Wow! Is that anywhere near here?" I ask.

"I've already checked the map, and it will only take us about forty minutes. If we leave a bit early we can even catch the sunrise!"

"You want to come, too?"

"Of course!" Eloise says. "I wouldn't miss it!"

I guess I shouldn't be surprised. Because we are motherless mothers and the best of friends, we do such things for one another often. Eloise once mentioned that her mom used to buy her a new warm nightgown for Christmas each year, so I ordered her a flannel dream from LL Bean. And Eloise always calls to see how my doctors' appointments go. Years ago, when I'd had my four wisdom teeth extracted, Eloise drove down to Manhattan.

When she came into our apartment I was moaning with pain, my cheeks puffed up like a chipmunk's.

"What are you giving her?" she asked Mitch.

"She had a Percodan a while ago, but she can't have another yet. I don't want her turning into a drug addict."

"Give me that bottle!" Eloise demanded. She shook out a pill, poured a glass of water, and handed it over to me, muttering, "Misguided man, hoarding those pills. What are you thinking?"

I've always loved Eloise for that, even though I got so high that their vitriolic arguments over the pros and cons of pain relievers rang in my ears like a Lucy/Ricky comedy skit.

Eloise and I stay up late talking, but in the morning we rise at 5 a.m. to watch the sunrise. (Sam comes with us, because he's the sort of kid who likes an adventure, but the rest of our boys— Aaron, Ben and Eloise's son Jeb —sleep in, as do our husbands.) We find an open shop where Eloise gets a coffee and Sam a doughnut. I order an egg on a croissant for some protein, and we settle on a bench by the dunes to watch the morning arrive.

"Let me take your picture!" Eloise cries at daybreak. "Stretch out your arm, holding your hand open!"

I follow Eloise's instruction and reach toward the sun. In the viewfinder, it appears that I'm cradling the glowing orb. This is how Eloise has always treated me; as if I *could* really hold the sun in my hands. From the day I first met Eloise, I've sensed only love and support from her, and that's just what I've given her back.

At seven, we scramble down the stairs to the beach, where I spot our teacher. As we approach, a slim older woman in sneakers and peddle pushers steps toward us.

"There are hundreds of seals just a twenty-minute walk down the shoreline!" she cries excitedly.

As Sam races off, I ask Eloise, only half-joking, "What if he's eaten by so many seals?"

"He traveled all the way to England; I think he can handle a walk up the beach," she grins.

We arrange our "mats" (today they're actually beach towels) and settle into the poses; as I move I'm aware that in this novice class I know what I'm doing. (I've reminded Eloise, who hasn't practiced yoga in twenty-five years and isn't exactly an exercise freak, about the challenges of certain postures.) I feel the breeze on my face, and seagulls soar overhead. I try to concentrate, but my mind wanders; I'm worried about Sam, even while knowing in my heart that he's fine.

The instructor guides us into Tree pose. For focus, we're to avoid looking at the water, or anything else that moves. As I struggle to maintain my balance, Sam appears, ambling across the beach directly in my line of vision, turning his head to grin sheepishly at me as he passes by. Against the teacher's advice, I follow his path with my gaze, and as I think back to the day he came safely home from abroad I topple joyously from my asana. As my feet dig into the sand to steady myself from falling flat on my face, I realize that Sam's trip to England was as important a step for me as it was for him. Finally, I've begun to fight back! Still, it's weird to be in a boxing match with myself, especially since I'm not really violent by nature.

My feet burrow into the sand. "Feel your body; feel your body against the sand, against the Earth. Notice the sensations," the teacher calls out, and I wish I could take her, the sand, the sun, the breeze, the water, the seals, the light, the gray, the salt air, this peace, and even Eloise back home with me. I wish I could bottle the sense of trust, so that whenever I feel unsure, I could just lift it to my nose and inhale.

We spend the days hiking, swimming and enjoying Eloise's seafood dinners, though our ocean swims are, as always for me, a little *too* exhilarating, and I can't bring myself to enter the water unless Mitch or the boys are near. My parents never took me to the ocean, and though I know some folks are squeamish about the fish and seaweed in a lake, I've always been more afraid of thrashing waves than a sunfish tickling my ankles. The first time I saw the ocean, I was about twelve; skinny little big-blue-eyed Beth had invited me to come to Maine on vacation with her family, and my parents allowed me to go, since Beth's dad was a physician and they always felt safe when I was with her (this couldn't have been further from the truth—Beth and I got into heaps of mischief, especially in our wily adolescent years). I was stunned by the extraordinary beauty of the ocean, and all that week, Beth and I held hands and dipped in and out of the waves.

Somewhere along the line, as with so many things in my life, my wariness metamorphosed into full-blown fear, and now I find it nearly impossible to enter the ocean without Mitch beside me. Today, however, he's fallen asleep under the umbrella, and I'm thirsting to feel the water on my skin. The boys have run off down the beach to search for "hot babes," and as I stand at the water's edge, I'm more like a woman in quicksand than one at the joyous entryway to the ocean. I imagine myself being sucked out to sea, lost in the eerie panic of trying to reach safety while the waves carry me further away. I wonder when my fear of the ocean became greater than my love of it.

I remember once at the lake, when I was just a toddler, wandering out onto a dock and clumsily slipping into the water. My mom was chatting with some elderly ladies on a bench nearby, and when she heard the splash she came running and snatched me up. The water was laden with fallen leaves, dark in the evening shadows, and I could feel my mother's chest pounding madly as she lifted me. I can *still* feel her heart beating with fear, so close to mine.

I turn back and plop down on the blanket next to Mitch. My husband can fall asleep anywhere, any time. Right now he's actually snoring, his lanky frame shaded by an umbrella, oblivious to the fact that he's totally missed my titillating Bay Watch moment!

We're back home, and when I wake up today, my stomach is roiling. Bright idea: I'll skip yoga! But this is Jill's class, and I missed last week, so I drag myself from bed; I'll just place myself in the rear of the studio and take it slow.

Only two people come to class today: a woman who's been practicing yoga for a decade and me. I have nowhere to hide, so I set my mat down in the center of the room, and the experienced yogini positions hers directly across from me. Jill tosses her shiny red hair and begins the class with the announcement that she's attended a very challenging yoga workshop, which she's going to share with us. We will learn to hold the poses longer than we thought possible by "going to the breath." Yoga is about the mind, she explains, but it's also about the postures. Jill instructs us to lunge forward and raise our arms in a Warrior pose. "Now," she says, "go deeper. And breathe."

I realize that we're re-enacting the lessons Jill has learned at her workshop, but can't she tell that if I go much deeper, I'll surely land on my ass?

Still, I find that I want to please her; I want her to believe that I'm as serious about yoga as she is, though I know that's not even possible. She seems to expect so much of us—but no more than she expects of herself.

I fear that I won't survive this class, yet by glancing at the other student now and then, and by thinking of my breath, I somehow muddle through. Yoga offers more than a few mixed messages; listen to your body vs. let your breath spirit you away from the urge to give up. Still, I've never been so happy to reach Savasana. I close my eyes, relax happily against my bolster, and breathe in the cool lavender scent of the eye pillow Jill places across my brow. Her warm hands knead my legs, as if they're dough for a piecrust, and pull at my outstretched arms, grounding my wandering thoughts.

Outside, trucks thrash up the road; I remember the sound of seagulls, the gentle caress of the ocean breeze.

I want so desperately to be content in the moment, but so often, the past and the future spirit the present away. I don't know why I feel more at home in my imagination than I do in reality, even when my imagination drags me deeper into my fears. It's almost as if I *choose* to be absent from the present.

I'm beginning to suspect that fear is something I don't have to live with—that I've *allowed* it to rule my life. But I have a right to change my mind; now I just need the tools and courage to do it. It's tricky, though, since the very qualities I need to fight back are those that I lack. I always have to laugh when I hear someone advise a child, "Don't be frightened!" What sane person would wake up in the morning and say, "Looks like a helluva great day for scaring the crap out of myself!"?

CHAPTER FOUR: SEPTEMBER

9/11 Fear of Flying to the Max

I can sense that summer is really ending when I walk to yoga tonight. The leaves are beginning to fall from our pear trees—they're always the first to go. I stand outside for a moment before heading down the hill, just surveying our tiny swatch of property. When we first moved in I had no idea how much I would come to love it, though the ivy trickling down the back door should have been a clue.

We'd planned to live here a year or two and then move on, but as with so many things, we soon became attached. I grew to love the cardinals and squirrels, the shabby little garage, the lilies of the valley that sprouted up under the Norway spruce, and of course, Anneke next door. No way were we leaving, so we borrowed money from relatives and the bank and turned our tiny new "mouse house" into a home that could accommodate three boys. The house is no longer fit for a mouse (although we've had a few come to visit). I take a last look and head down the block.

Tonight, Ali, my first yoga teacher, is back from her trip to France. "I hope you've all been practicing on your own," she says. "Even five minutes a day is better than nothing!" She sits in Lotus position at the front of the room, staring intensely at each of us. As always, I feel that her dark, searching gaze rests longer on me, as if she expects more of me than the others (maybe because I'm older, and more out of shape?). Ali laughs often, but not in a light-hearted way. I don't exactly feel that she's laughing *at* us, but she's not really laughing *with* us either. It seems as if she's laughing at something she knows inside; something that we can't yet fathom.

I've not forgotten how demanding Ali can be, even though she speaks softly. She leads us through a lovely sequence. After a few rounds, she tells us to continue independently at our own pace. With my peripheral vision, I copy the movements of the others; my own mind vacant, like a dyslexic child in a classroom of fluent readers. I am yoga disabled, apparently, for I can't remember which pose comes next without the voice of an instructor to guide me. I think of how kindly my friend Anneke spoke to a frightened little boy on the diving board at the town pool one day; I wish she were here now to help me through this, to reassure me that I can do it, that I am capable and strong. I seem to need to hear these words from someone else, since I can't possibly say them to myself with conviction.

I notice that the only other woman in the class who appears to be near fifty is also having difficulty. She knows what pose comes next, but can't balance. I'm ashamed to admit that her failure pleases me; I'm mentally handicapped, perhaps, but my balance is still relatively intact! To her right is a young woman who is as tall as the Mountain pose, with a long braid down her back and slim, graceful arms and fingers. In the rear of the studio a young black woman moves with precision; she turns and sways into her poses like a dancer. I realize I'm beginning to know these women, to recognize them by the sounds of their breath, by the tenor of their "Om" at the beginning and end of class. Occasionally, we take partners, helping one another with our poses, beginning to know one another through our own bodies, in ways we can't with our neighbors at home.

Apart from childbirth and sex, nothing has touched my body like yoga. This must be what conventional sports are to some women; the stretch of an arm as one serves a tennis ball, or the flex of the thighs before a dive, must offer the athlete the same familiar sense of knowledge and companionship I'm beginning to recognize when I come to yoga.

After class, Ali says we won't be meeting next week. Sighs of disappointment follow her announcement, and as we leave, we share our concerns. We've come to *need* yoga now— like water, sleep, or a slice of first-rate pizza. How strange to be craving something that I took half a century to try.

It's dark now when I walk up my hill. Mitch is waiting for me outside the door, a worried frown on his face. He's a very devoted husband, perhaps too much so. Music is his "other life," but when it comes to close friends, I'm his one and only (he doesn't like to shoot hoops or drink beer with the guys). My husband demands a lot of me, and sometimes there's no way I can live up to his expectations. And I suspect that he's slightly jealous of my newfound love of yoga, because it's taking up more and more of the time I might be spending with him.

"Are you okay?" he asks as I come closer.

"Of course."

He places his arm around my shoulder, and we stand together, gazing up the street. When the boys were younger we spent hours watching them ride their bikes on this quiet little dead end stretch of cement. At times, I sense that Mitch and I are remembering the same scenes from our life together, even though we don't always say so. I feel that way tonight.

Yes, it's nice to know he cares about me, but I just want to be alone, especially after yoga class, which takes me far away, to a place in my own center. Maybe this longing for solitude is a good thing, since one day my children will be grown and gone. I fear that impending time as much as I've ever feared anything; when I imagine their empty beds and rooms, I feel that familiar panic in my heart, that fear of leaving and letting go. I *wish* I could be the mother who follows the words of Kahlil Gibran—bravely sending my children out into the world like "living arrows," holding firm like the sturdy bow. But instead *I* am the quiver— the quivering mess, that is.

I wonder if yoga will help me face my child-less reality when it arrives. If Aaron's departure for college and Sam's trip to England were the warm-ups, I can only imagine the sleepless nights, and the doom and despair that will rise from my heart as I prepare to send my last two sons off. Here I go again, imagining the future, imagining the worst, feeding with my thoughts the very fears that make me so unhappy. Saying good-bye is harder than childbirth in some ways; painful as it was, at least that was a, "Hey, kiddo, *hello*."

Back to school week is here. Aaron has driven his own car back for his senior year of college, and Sam and Ben are both in high school. I don't have to hold their hands and walk them to elementary school anymore, though I still have to make those hateful bag lunches in the morning. I figure I've made thousands of these suckers, and the tedium can be exhausting, since they'll only eat turkey or ham on white bread or cream cheese on a bagel. Anything green or crunchy (lettuce, tomatoes, onions) or any suspicious spread (pesto, mustard or mayo) is immediately and vehemently rejected. Since birth, they've been picky eaters, even though I've followed the parenting rulebook, "offering" everything from tofu to asparagus.

Sometimes, when I'm slapping these sandwiches together in the morning, it strikes me that I've spent a heck of a lot of years trying to please these little males that surround me (not to mention the big one). I've been here almost every day for them after school (no latchkey kids in this family), I've attended all their concerts and ballgames, helped them with homework every night, and done everything possible to have a family dinner on the table at least five nights out of seven. And the payoffs have been grand. We've raised three kind-hearted, intelligent kids who love us and adore one another. Other than quite a few fistfights (sort of like the Bonanza boys), speeding tickets, and broken bones they've been marvelous children, and I don't for an instant wish I'd worked more, or longer, or sent them all away to Hogwarts. But at times, I do wonder where has the time gone? It's as if the clock has fast-forwarded twenty years in the blink of an eye, and now I'm wondering exactly what am I to do without the bag lunches, without the homework hours, without the lessons and ballgames and carpooling? How am I—now over fifty—supposed to reclaim my life? I feel as if I've spent the past two decades working on a huge, grand family canvas, and now the painting is nearly completed. My creation is awesomely beautiful, but how am I to top it?

Of course, now that summer's over and there are no teenagers sleeping till noon and then straggling into the kitchen for breakfast, my daytime hours are my own, though Mitch is always looking to take a walk or spend some quiet time together when he doesn't have a morning rehearsal. As much as I love to be with him, I'm not available on my yoga mornings. I'm pursuing this new pastime with nearly compulsive dedication, in part, I think, because I so much want to "catch up" with the others, even though I know that's really not possible; no matter how much I learn, they'll always be Handstands ahead of me.

Once again, I'm yoga challenged. When Jill says to place our right arm across our left elbow, I do the opposite. When she says to bend right, I bend to the left. Jill notices and says, "*You* bend to the right now." I laugh, not really caring, and she smiles back at me, in a way that tells me she notices exactly where I am in my practice. Somehow, I feel that she's waiting for me to catch up to something, for me to "get it." This isn't just about Handstands—it has to do with where I am in life. Yet it seems as if she's reaching out her hand, as if she believes I'll arrive in time. I wish I were as hopeful about my progress as Jill seems to be.

At the end of class, some of the women do Headstands. I opt for a Handstand prep—my feet high on the wall behind me. Surprisingly, my hips lift up without much cajoling. My arms shake weakly, yet I hold the pose. "It's not about the poses," Jill has said. "It *is* about the poses," she's said, too. It's all so damn confounding!

In a class that teaches nonattachment, one of the primary tenets of yoga philosophy, I'm becoming attached to Jill and Ali, but this just seems to be my nature. I enjoy Jill's classes so much, even when they're strenuous. She always starts with an introductory lesson or a bit of Buddhist philosophy; she makes the class an intimate, private conversation.

In Ali's class (I've come to call her "the Gestapo lady"), the poses sometimes feel like punishments, as if she's getting satisfaction from our suffering. I'm sure that's not true; it's just the way I feel while holding the Downward Dog pose for five long breaths. It's important, it seems, to like one's yoga teacher, but it may be even better if at times you detest her, too.

∞

I do yoga on my own for a few minutes this morning. I'm learning to slow down a bit, and I notice the desire to practice yoga is replacing some of my more negative wishes; sometimes, I think of practicing yoga instead of having a cigarette, for instance. I gave up smoking years ago, but if a smoker is nearby I still often feel the temptation.

I'm reading a book about yoga, and the author, Geeta Iyengar, says, "Women need yoga even more than men as the responsibilities thrust upon them by Nature are greater than men's." I'm not sure what that means, exactly, since men, by nature, are forced into roles of warrior and provider. But women give birth to children, and maybe doing for others *is* a more strenuous type of battle.

On the way to class this evening, I glance up at the darkening sky; the clouds are luminous blue and gray, and the moon is a perfect half. Tonight Ali joins us in the asanas, and she's unusually gentle. Either she's holding the poses for less time, or I'm more accustomed to them. She teaches a new pose called "Half Moon" and I'm astounded.

"We'll do Shoulderstand now," Ali says, helping us arrange blankets. We lift up our hips, our weight on our upper backs and shoulders. As we hold, she tells us that the word Buddha means "awake."

"We too, can be Buddhas; we too, can be awake," Ali claims.

I like the idea that I can still open my eyes and learn at my age. I also like the idea that I'm getting stronger and less afraid to press my body into "taffy." I doubt that I'll ever do a Headstand or Handstand, but maybe it's not out of the realm of possibility. A few months ago, I'd have doubled over with laughter at the mere suggestion.

After class I approach Ali. "There's a half moon outside; did you see it?"

"You're kidding!" she cries. We stand grinning at one another, as if we're two scientists in a lab who've just made a fabulous discovery.

As I walk home beneath the moon and stars, I feel a certain pleasure in the knowledge that tonight I've imitated nature. It almost feels as if the moon is sending a magnetic lightness to my footsteps, guiding me calmly and evenly along my path.

Sun pours in my windows on this late-September morning, and I awaken at 6 a.m. I've tossed from my side to my back to the other side to my stomach a hundred times in the past hour. My mind races; for some reason, I've chosen this morning to ruminate about sending Sam to college. We have two years, yet *this* is the morning I've decided to obsess about the impending departure of my middle child: Where will he go? What will he major in? How will I say good-bye and actually drive away? Maybe the shrink *does* have something I could pop for this one: the College Prep morning *before* pill for moms, instead of the morning after?

Of course, part of the reason I'm so terrified of the day Sam will leave is because of what happened on the day Aaron left. It was during the two hours that I was fluffing Aaron's pillow in his freshman dorm room and helping him unpack his clothes that my mother died. I had chosen to be with my son in southern Jersey, thinking I'd make it back to upstate New York in plenty of time to sit by my mother's bedside. And even though I know my mother would have forgiven me for making that choice— *Forgive?* My generous, selfless mom would never have wanted me to miss my son's first day of college; au contraire, she insisted from her deathbed that I accompany Aaron— still, I've never forgiven *myself.* Nor have I ever gotten past the horrific events that occurred just two weeks after my mother died—9/11 and its aftermath, when my personal world and the world at large came crashing down simultaneously.

Yoga is about nurturing the self, and I suspect this is one of its main draws. I've always been uncomfortable with the "sinner" aspect of Christianity. I prefer to think we are little lambs who have lost our way (baa, baa, baa) and the yogis seem to promote that sentiment. It's okay to be kind to ourselves. It's okay to forgive.

∞

Tonight, we seem to frustrate Ali; she frowns when none of us can negotiate a new posture, which she calls "Crow." She *looks* like a crow as she demonstrates; her thick black hair like feathers as she places her hands on her mat, raises her hips and balances on her arms. We all attempt, but none of us succeeds. I'm sure if I balance my head on the block, as she suggests, my brains will spill onto the floor.

I'm beginning to think that some of the yoga teachers see their students as reflections of their own success or failure. I want to tell Ali that she's a fantastic teacher, whether or not we can do the "Crow." It's quite possible to give all the right directions and encouragement and still be unable to teach the posture to someone who isn't quite ready to learn. I want to remind her that just three months ago Downward Dog was a torturous punishment for me, while now that once loathsome asana is actually a cakewalk.

When I come in from class, Sam stops me in my tracks. "I don't want to live here anymore," he announces. "Now that I've been to England, this little town seems stupid. School is a waste of my time."

"Oh, Sam," I sigh. "There are plenty of positives about our town and school. You just need some time to readjust."

"Well, *I* can't see any," Sam snaps, closing his door.

I hesitate outside. How to explain that opening up the world shouldn't diminish the value of everyday life? Sam is sixteen, and like the yoginis tonight, perhaps not ready to learn this lesson. At least he's learned the extraordinary value of travel and opening one's self to new experiences; now he must acknowledge the counterpart— that treasuring the familiar is also important in life. I know this lesson very well; it's the reverse *I* have yet to master.

I'm glad I have one child left who seems to still like it here. In fact, I can't get Ben to come out of his room. He's so hooked into his computer that it's beginning to worry me, though Aaron was the same at his age, and simply ended up a computer science major. It's hard to believe that for years Ben and I were connected at the hip. He was the one baby who received my undivided attention—by the time I had him at age thirty-eight, I was winding down my magazine writing, concentrating on smaller local assignments. I'd waved the white flag to motherhood by then, so Ben and I spent days together taking walks and reading (it was a voluntary surrender, despite my mixed emotions). I'd made a commitment by then to the marriage, too. I know you're supposed to do this on your wedding day, but my matrimonial hormones didn't kick in with the exchange of vows. My heart told me I was marrying the *right* guy, but it also warned, "This ain't gonna be easy, Honey."

Though Aaron and Sam may have heard their parents bickering about roles and careers a bit more than was healthy, happily for Ben the marriage was firm as he was growing up, and he seems to be a reflection of that devotion. Though he spends a lot of time online like any teenager, Ben's a witty writer and has plenty of friends; with his wiry frame and curly hair he often reminds me of Mitch when I first met him. I view all my kids as wondrous in their own right, but also as grand, miraculous rewards I've received just for hanging in there. Mitch always said that if there were a God in Heaven, all my babies would be boys.

He meant that as a threat, but it's actually been a blessing.

Growing into womanhood in the braless Seventies, I developed the attitude that men were callous at their worst, or at their best, emotionally clueless. Becoming the mother of sons taught me that little boys have feelings and tears, that they harbor sadness and worries, that they're capable of astonishing moments of humor and insight; and it taught me that these miraculous baby boys grow into young men who still have these qualities, who still cry, and bleed both physically and spiritually. If I'd had daughters, I'd have had a different kind of love in my life, but Mitch was so right—I gave birth to the children I needed. My guess is that we *all* do.

Pumping Iron, Pressing the Panic Button

I'm having a week of mysterious aches, and I'm wondering if this has anything to do with the fact that I've missed a few yoga classes. I tried pulling out my mat one day, but after a few minutes of stretching, I had a shooting pain in my lower back. Quite possibly, I don't know what the hell I'm doing.

My thoughts relax when Ali begins. The mat is soft and welcoming beneath my stiff body, and as we bend and stretch, I feel as if I've come home. It's odd that a slim purple mat can seem like a lifeboat. As we rise and try what Ali calls the "Dancer's Pose" I'm amazed that I can actually hold one foot behind me and lean forward.

Even after a week off my mat, I'm balancing! I realize that yoga is all about balance: the balance of mind, body, and spirit, the balance of bending into a pose that seems unattainable until one tries. Most of my troubles have been about balance, after all; family and career, self and others, balancing love, balancing fear. I've let so many things pull me in so many directions—I need to find a way to embrace the whole of life without collapsing.

∞

At 4 a.m., I awaken with my heart pounding wildly, and I sit straight up in bed. I feel as if the doom of the world is resting on my shoulders, and my left arm is numb and tingling. With the history of heart attacks in my family, I can't help thinking that I may be having one. Or maybe it's some kind of panic attack.

I throw off my covers and lower myself onto my bedroom floor. I'm burning up: perhaps this is just one mother of a menopausal hot flash! I can imagine the emergency technicians having a real guffaw over that. Of course, thinking about what the EMTs might say is fairly idiotic.

Mitch is away with the ballet in Los Angeles, so I'm here with the kids alone. The thought of them waking up to an ambulance siren isn't attractive, and even though they're much older than I was when my dad was carted away, I don't especially want to relive that scenario.

I grab a medical book off a nearby shelf, pad into the bathroom for a glass of water, and settle in on my floor by my bed again, flipping through the pages and sipping the cool water. I try to take deep breaths and focus, but my heart is racing. What in the world is this all about?

It's 5 o'clock in the morning but I decide to phone my doctor. Apparently, he doesn't think I'm in dire danger, since he suggests I drop by the office at ten. I crawl back into bed, hoping I don't wake up in Heaven (or Hell!), kicking myself for not dialing 911. I toss and turn, trying to figure out where this is coming from. My mother never had panic attacks to my knowledge, but then my mother rarely forced herself outside her comfort zone. She didn't ride on subways or go to work outside the home, and she didn't live in highway-crazed New Jersey. My father never traveled, and until the day he died, she was never really alone. But maybe that's the difference; I have all my mother's fears and then some, but I've summoned mine forth for a duel. Unlike Mom, I don't want to spend my life in a five-bedroom Victorian house, driving only to the grocery store. (Okay, I'd like the five-bedroom Victorian house, but I'd want it to be home base— not a prison— and it would have to be close to Manhattan.)

I breathe more slowly, and finally fall back asleep. When I awaken again, the sun is shining, and I feel splendid; I get the kids up for school, take a shower, and head over to my internist's office.

"What's the problem?" asks the nurse as she checks my vitals.

"I don't really know. I woke up in the middle of the night convinced I was going to die. I never felt so horrible in my life! Well, except for three other times, maybe. But there was an obvious symptom: my belly was the size of a watermelon."

The nurse nods as if she's already heard this complaint a hundred times today, and maybe she has. I know I'm not alone in my anxiety issues; half the world seems to be on anti-depressants or anti-anxiety meds these days. She ushers me into an inner office and leaves me to sit fidgeting until my doctor finally opens the door.

"Hop up on the examining table!" my internist says cheerily (maybe he's on antidepressants himself!). He pokes and prods, discovering a mysterious bite on my belly. "I'll run a test for Lyme disease, but most likely you've just had a panic attack." He steps out of the examining room, presumably to order the blood test.

The nurse rolls in with an EKG machine; I won't be surprised if she finds an irregularity. But my EKG is normal, my internist says when he comes back in to check the results, and he's not concerned about my heart. Maybe it's my "other" heart that I should be worried about, the one deep within that's so connected to my husband.

The rest of the day is uneventful, and in the crisp autumn night I walk to class where Ali tells us to "let go." I wonder what the difference is between letting go and falling over. As I stand in Mountain pose, I sway as if I've just downed four Margaritas. I can't find the middle of my pose, can't ground myself. When we stand in Tadasana—which is, really, just standing straight, after all—I have the funniest feeling. My feet are so firmly planted on my mat, and yet when I close my eyes, I have the sensation that I'm about to fall. Standing straight and strong on a mat, I feel less balanced than I do just walking down the sidewalk. Being aware of where I am in life is enough to make me keel over!

Maybe, like my mother, I really *am* just afraid of being alone. Certainly, I'm disappointed that after four months of yoga, I've behaved this way. Mitch says that people who do yoga won't die at my age. If that's true, then I can't figure out why this panic attack occurred. Maybe I expect too much of yoga, as if I think it will save my life. Weird, but it almost seems as if my body is trying to send me a telegram. A child development expert I once interviewed claimed that when children throw tantrums or act out, they're just trying to give their parents a message.

"Are you *listening*?" the psychologist would ask.

∞

Two days later, I'm back at Jill's class; she's relentless this morning, tossing her hair and flexing her muscles. I keep glancing at the clock in the corner, wishing the class were over.

"It's a new moon," Jill observes, "and we should all think about objectives we want to accomplish in the coming year."

The only thing I can think of is maintaining good health. I hope I don't get sick and that my family stays healthy, too. The other night's experience— panic attack or whatever— has made me realize that there's nothing more precious than health. This is another reason why yoga is so important. It's part of my quest to gain back control of my body after so many years of treating it poorly.

Jill places her hands on the floor, tips forward, and lifts her hips so that her body rests on her elbows. This is "Crow pose" again, and I already know that I can't do it. I topple to the side repeatedly as she scolds, "Crows don't hop!"

Maybe crows don't hop, but I'll bet plenty of other birds do, I think to myself combatively.

"It will come when you're ready," she assures me, as if she can read my mind.

At last we rest in Savasana, and I feel Jill's gentle hands pull at my arms. "Whatever you give out you will receive ten-fold," she whispers soothingly. "If you want love, give love."

I squeeze my eyes more tightly shut in wonder. I'm not sure whether I *do* want more love in my life or whether it's the very wealth of love that has caused me so many problems. At the very least, it's losing love that's at the core of my fear. And anyway, no matter how much love I give out, I can't have my mother back.

When I arrive at yoga class today, several students are discussing their fingernail polish. Next, they chat about their plans for the weekend. Many of the ladies who come to class seem to have money; yoga sure isn't a poor woman's pursuit in America.

Within a few moments, our yoga room is filled to capacity, and everyone seems to know one another. These are the "power yoginis," and for some reason, they intimidate me profoundly today. I find myself forcing to maintain the poses to impress these women, wondering if they notice how unbalanced and unfocused I am. Before class, I discovered that my shirt was on inside out. Thank God I saw the tag at my neck in the mirror! I've always had a horrible fear of showing up in the wrong kind of clothing, but I never thought I'd experience this at yoga class.

Not surprisingly, witchy little Jill's focus today is on how we need to value ourselves. "Think about how great you are!" Jill instructs as she travels around the room adjusting our poses, placing her hands lightly on our hips or shoulders. "Don't dwell on your faults; think about what a perfect, amazing person you are."

I feel as if I'm the only woman here who has nothing especially redeeming to claim as my accomplishments. They're all expertly manicured, shapely, and in control of their bodies. I bet not a one would smoke a cigarette or drink too much chardonnay. I doubt any would use the F word around their children. I recall the time when the boys were little and I lost it and called them "fucker shits." For weeks, they echoed the phrase like a trio of cackling parrots, thrilled to rat me out to Mitch and anyone else they encountered, including little old ladies at the grocery store. They even told my *Mom.*

"Mommy called us fucker shits!" Sam announced proudly.

"*Kathy!*" my mother gasped.

It's a cool, late October evening and in yoga class, we practice something called ujjayi breathing, a technique in which you narrow your vocal chords so you sound a little like Deep Throat. Normally, I *pretend* I'm doing a breathing method when I'm not, but tonight Ali steps around the room, listening to determine if we're practicing correctly, bending close and tapping her foot until we do it right. My breath sounds like a conch shell at the ocean, so she says I pass muster. I find it difficult to think about the way I breathe; almost impossible. Mitch says he notices I often hold my breath;

sometimes he wonders if I've just stopped breathing altogether. But yoga is changing that, and I can sense the feeling of peace that comes when you stop and pay attention. Mitch is acutely aware of the breath, being a wind player. Perhaps that's why he's such a calm, centered presence—the exact opposite of me. In many ways we're oil and water, but of course, opposites attract.

"I have a question for you," Ali says. "What have you gained from yoga?"

We go around the class, each of us offering our thoughts. Some say "peace," others say "balance." For once, I speak up, without hesitation: "A clear space for my mind, a time to flee from my worries and anxieties."

When I'm in yoga class, I don't think about Sam going off to college in a year, or where Aaron will get a job when he graduates, or whether Ben is growing up too fast, or what the hell I'm going to do with the rest of my life when my children are gone. I am here now, and for a brief hour or so, my other life vanishes. When I'm in yoga class, it's as if I kick my fears off outside the door with my shoes. Yes, I pick them back up when I leave, but they do seem lighter for a while.

The presidential election approaches, and I've been staying up later and later, listening to liberal talk radio, tooling around the Internet, sipping wine and ruminating about the state of the country. Anneke and I get together often to talk about politics; Mitch and I constantly banter about Kerry and Bush and the Iraq war, and sometimes I think all this worrying about the future of America isn't good for me. Yoga seems a calm respite from the tension, yet I wonder whether hiding my head between my legs is really the best solution. Maybe I should be out picketing instead.

I'm rather glad October is almost over. I love the crisp, cool nights and the swirling leaves, but the season also reminds me of the night my father died sixteen years ago, alone, in a hospital room. My mom and Ruthann had gone home for the night, expecting Dad would be released in the morning, but instead, he didn't make it. I had seen Dad a week or so before, and though I suspected he wasn't long for this world, I had planned to drive up from Jersey and visit again. In any case, my last words to him were "I love you." My mother always lamented the fact that she never said a proper good-bye, as if you could say a final good-bye to someone you'd been married to for half a century.

As a child, I'd wait with anticipation for my dad to come home from the courthouse, pulling into the drive in his pointy-finned white Chrysler. He'd push me on a homemade swing while he smoked his pipe. My dad loved to fish, and I swear he loved worms. He used to itch for a rainy summer night so he could step out into the darkness with an empty bucket. I'd follow in my nightgown and sneakers with a flashlight. "Shine the light over here!" he'd order. "Ah hah! A big one!" He'd pull out the long, brown night crawler from the dark, cold grass and pop it triumphantly into the pail.

The next morning he'd be up at 5:30; maybe it wasn't the fish he was after so much as just the opportunity to be a grown man playing with worms, because when I went along, he didn't get to do much fishing. Instead, he'd spend the dawn curling worms on my fish hooks, throwing in my line and helping me get untangled when it landed in the rocks or weeds. Those worms would wriggle around his thick fingers, and once in a while I'd reach over and touch. They felt otherworldly; things I didn't want to know about. My dad had such patience, his own line sitting abandoned on the side of the boat. Sometimes, he'd see it pull and he'd snatch up his rod and reel in a small-mouth bass. I was in awe; I hated the worms, but I loved to sit with my father on a still, silent lake, leaning every now and then to touch the bright mustard cup of a lily pad. Out

on the lake life was so simple: my father hooked the worms and—
for a brief few hours— I felt safe.

Yet Another Lost Election

Today is the election; I pry myself away from the television, cast my vote in the gym at the boys' school, and head to yoga. Silently, I dedicate my practice to John Kerry. Silly goose that I am, I've been hoping for months that America will choose the path of the peaceful warrior.

Ali seems to lack patience with us tonight. My "Crow" doesn't take flight, nor does my Handstand prep. Ali sighs; she seems to have no interest in helping me, and visibly controls an urge to criticize. I usually sense calmness from Ali, but tonight she's on edge. Maybe she's rooting for Kerry, too.

I suppose it doesn't help that half of my friends are Republicans, which is a zany thing. It's not as if I went out and tracked down pals who are my exact political opposite, but like so much in my life—and in yoga—opposing energies seem to attract. I belong to a "wine tasting club," for instance, that is mostly right-wingers ("tasting," here, is a bit of a euphemism). A dozen of us became friends after working together on a school referendum, discovering only later that while we all adore wine, we're in grave opposition when it comes to the national political landscape. Still, when I'm with these friends—as long as we don't talk Bush —we're filled with laughter and fun. One of them—Billy—is a Vietnam vet who believes that there is a God because "there *has* to be," which I think is as good a reason as I've ever heard. I love this guy completely, and his wife, Annie, too. Thankfully, I also have a lot of liberal friends. I have a lot of friends, period, perhaps because I need them to vent with when living with boys and a musician husband becomes too intense. Or maybe, because I just love having friends. I've cultivated these friendships devotedly; I carry the sorrows and problems of my friends like rocks in my pockets.

Sometimes I feel like a starfish with my arms reaching out, but I have many more friends than a starfish has arms, and I suspect there must be a reason. My mom never had any friends outside our family; she didn't do lunch or coffee with anyone other than my dad or my aunts or grandma. There was no Eloise, Anneke or Beth in her life, and I always thought it both beautiful and sad to see her waiting by the window for my father to come home.

As much as I admire my mother's generosity and kindness, I'd like to take my version of her to the next level. Yes, I'm my mother's daughter, but I also want to learn how to tap into my own strength, my own heart.

Mitch has raced out to sub at Phantom (I love it when he dresses all in black for this gig, like a clarinet-wielding Zorro), the boys are on their computers, and I'm off to Ali's class. We're meeting again in the whimsical children's room. Ali decides to hover near me; often she seems to pick out one student, upon whom she bestows added attention for a night. She follows my movements, gently stretching my arms higher, kneading my clenched shoulders as we rest with our backs arched over bolsters. I don't like massages, or to have my fingernails painted in a salon, so Ali's touch is somewhat alarming. All the yoga instructors touch their students—some, more than others, but so far, I've managed to escape prolonged physical contact.

Tonight, I'm trapped, but decide to "go with the flow." I'd *like* to be a woman who goes for massages, facials and pedicures… but so far I'm not. I "do" my own toes, henna my own hair, and have even been known to cut my own bangs (big mistake!).

I'm reminded of a weekend excursion I attended with my book club. Six of us spent a night at a classy hotel; we went out to dinner, stayed up drinking and laughing, and slept in queen-sized beds together like little girls. In the morning, most of the women went to the spa for massages and facials, but I headed home. They thought it was incredibly silly that I refused to have my feet or neck rubbed by a stranger. But my mother was just like this; she never had her nails or hair professionally done her entire life, never spent a night away from her family with girlfriends, never sat up till 2 a.m. drinking wine. She's both the person from whom I learned to give love freely and from whom I learned how to hold back.

As a role model, my mother was a mix of positive and negative qualities. She spent her days dusting (I was fascinated by dust as a child), ironing, washing the clothes, and in the afternoon, watching her favorite soap on TV. Her main gig over the years was as family caregiver; she cared for everyone with phone calls and cards, hot meals, and an open invitation to visit. My mother was afraid of no person's problem and she never judged. She accepted all races, religions, sexual persuasions, political affiliations, shapes and sizes. This enormous capacity for love was counterbalanced by her fears, and she served both her love and her warnings like an elaborate buffet. My mother never had a nasty word to say about anyone, though occasionally I caught her rolling her eyes. The worst I ever heard her utter was that so-and-so was "a little *snooty*!" She never used a swear word in her life (though she wasn't a prude!) and she cringed when I'd get going.

Ali is firmly rubbing my neck; she's a very sensual teacher. All the teachers have curvaceous bodies, with tattoos and firm, supple skin; yoga seems to mold the body in a mysterious way that's muscular but feminine. I'd like to think that *my* body is changing, and from the feel of my clothes, I think that it is. I do feel stronger than when I began, even though I was six months younger then, but this newfound strength isn't just in my muscles; I'm beginning to sense that yoga reaches deep, to a place within that can't even be located anatomically.

November is settling in; opera season is coming to a close, and soon Mitch will be home more, unless he's called to sub at the ballet, where the clarinetists each year seem to come down with perplexing illnesses apparently related to playing too many Nutcrackers, as if the Sugar Plum Fairy delights in sprinkling flu germs.

I walk to the studio and settle into its warmth, though once we get moving I wonder if I'll pass out. I understand there are centers where people do yoga in extreme heat. (I doubt the participants are menopausal and already burning up like I am!) Jill squeezes my shoulders and I realize my neck is unbearably tight; it's amazing how inflexible I become in between classes. I know I should practice more at home, cut back on the chardonnay, drink more water....

Enough picking on myself; so anti-yoga! "Let your aura shine," one of my classmates advised before class when I mentioned I'm worried about where this country is heading. Perhaps it's possible to become so immersed in yoga that you no longer focus on what's happening in the outside world. That might be good for me. After all, I've been obsessing about a draft lately; imagine being the mother of three sons now with the Iraq War raging. A single letter from the government could destroy the fabric of my life, and this makes me realize how unpredictable my seemingly structured existence really is. Maybe part of the joy of yoga comes from being able to control one's body in a world in which you can't control anything else. That ol' Iceberg Theory again. I can't seem to shake it.

I'm reminded today that I've become complacent, even in yoga. I haven't been pushing myself. The class is no more difficult than usual, but simple poses that I feel I've mastered seem impossible. This is what it all means, perhaps. Simple things in life, too, can suddenly become complex and unmanageable, just the way a marriage can seem one day perfect and the next in shambles, or I can feel one day that I'm totally on top of my children's progress, and the next conclude that I've slipped up horribly.

My writers' group seems to be floundering, too. We meet this afternoon, as we do every couple of weeks. We gather around a table at one of our homes with cups of coffee, holding our unfinished manuscripts. Jessica, a witty thirty-two-year-old, chatters about her kids; pretty Kayla, also in her thirties, discusses her house décor and Amy, who is my age, is fretting about her job as a newspaper editor. I sit sulking, wondering when we're going to sell our writing. And even though we adore each other and love to sit together trading stories, we're just treading water. We should each be writing our hearts out, and we know it.

I love that we're various ages, at different stages of life; I love these women, and yet they frustrate me, and I'm impatient because they keep veering off track. But right now they're raising children, nesting in their homes, contributing financially to their families. We're all in different places in our lives, just as the yoginis are on their mats. I gaze around the table, appreciating Jessica's sparkling blue eyes, Kayla's contagious, melodic laughter, Amy's soft, earnest expression. Suddenly, something inside is telling me to *stop* pushing and rushing, and expecting others to do the same.

∞

The Thanksgiving holiday is over! We went to my sister-in-law's; for the first time since my mother died, we celebrated the holiday with my husband's side of the family instead of mine. Some of the guests were conservatives; to counteract the toxins, I drank like a fish and ended up in a dreadful argument with an undercover cop wearing a thick gold cross around his neck. It was all about war and his contention that I should be just tickled pink to send my teenaged sons off to defend their country. I *know* I drank too much because I ended up blubbering on my mother-in-law's shoulder (though she doesn't imbibe, she didn't mind because she's a peacenik herself).

I wake up today feeling fat and hung-over. I trudge through the day, still livid whenever I think of that man's tirade, still feeling the effects of too much wine, too much food, and too many negative thoughts. So yoga, on this late November evening, seems like nirvana. The studio is a heavenly place of chimes, chants and the scent of lavender. This place—which so frightened me with its unfamiliarity the first time I entered—has become a safe haven. No one here will tell me to send my boys to war—no one here will tell me it's right to harm a fly. One woman describes her own vegetarian Thanksgiving. These people don't want to kill a freaking *turkey*!

Ali begins the session with a meditation. We sit silently and close our eyes. We're to think as little as possible, to accept our thoughts and then send them away into the silence. When we open our eyes three minutes later, it seems as if an eternity has passed. Ali tells us that we should use meditation in our lives, and it occurs to me that if I could do that, my life would seem much longer. No wonder the ancient yogis sat for hours in caves just meditating their little hearts out!

The poses are so welcomed tonight. I'm happy to remember I have legs and arms and a back that can stretch and ten functioning toes. I've spent the past week without my body, totally caught up in my worries about war and Thanksgiving and family and what will become of our country, to the point that I don't even know I *have* a body any more (other than to abuse, by eating and drinking too much).

Yoga is a strange companion. Now that I know what it's like to be away from it, I realize I actually *yearn* for yoga. As I glance at the faces of the other women in my classes, I know that they're searching for answers, too.

Message from a Butterfly

Christmas is coming, the geese are getting fat…and I've been scurrying from store to store trying to get a package together to send to my sister and her family in North Carolina: it's that scurrying time of year, and yoga is the perfect antidote.

Today Jill reminds, "Nothing stays the same forever, so try not to be so attached." Things may seem horrible now, and next week sublime, or vice versa. Maybe part of the appeal of yoga is that it *is* the same; the same breath, the same Downward Dog. But then again, it's never *exactly* the same. Sometimes the poses affect me in different ways, and what seems taxing today may seem simple next time, or the reverse. There's comfort in the familiarity of the poses (once you get to know them), but you never take the pose in precisely the same manner. My Tree is wobbling today, for instance, while last week I stood straight.

I take a Child's pose and Jill massages my back, as if to let me know it's all right; I don't always have to push myself. Part of what I need from yoga is the pushing, part the serenity and acceptance. Still, I'm surprised, in a way, that I'm still here. It's almost a compulsion, but one that's good for me. The little voice inside my head that cries, "This is too hard for you...just quit!" is drowned out by the deeper, wiser, yoga voice that says, "Just keep going." It's sort of like the muse I hear when I'm writing.

When I arrive home, Mitch is waiting to go out to lunch. As we walk toward the center of town, I consider what a curious life I'm living. Most of my friends spend time with their husbands on weekends while mine is working until midnight. But on weekdays, we spend hours walking, stopping for an inexpensive lunch, sitting on our deck sipping coffee and watching the birds. Because I'm a freelancer, I don't have to show up at an office. When the kids were young and required bedtime stories and baths, I cursed the fact that Mitch worked nights and weekends; but now, in my middle age, his is the perfect schedule. This, I realize, is one good thing about aging; as your children grow, your time becomes your own again, and you're old enough to know how to spend it wisely.

It's odd that I'm thinking about this because tonight— inspired by a silly TV show—Ben asks me to recount once again how I met his father. I was a junior, all of sixteen, sitting in the back row of chemistry class when a new boy came in. This in itself was peculiar, since you don't usually get transfers that late in the high school game. But this guy was not only a senior, he was cute; it turned out his parents had bought a new house on my side of town over the summer.

Unfortunately, he looked like a "freak," a term we used in those days for hard-core hippies. He had long, curly black hair and his body was so skinny and taut I decided he must be on Speed. At the very least he was surely a pothead, and though my current boyfriend smoked plenty of pot, I didn't need a guy in my life who might be doing harder drugs.

He was awfully attractive though, and within ten minutes he'd decided to fix his gaze on me, even though he was seated in the front row and had to twist his neck 180 degrees.

After class, when I was standing with my girlfriend next to the Bunsen burners, he sauntered over and boldly asked, "Would you be my lab partner?"

"I already have one," I smiled. My friend and I giggled as he walked away.

Though from time to time he'd call me, we didn't really connect again in high school. Mitch dropped out of chemistry (he convinced the administrators it was an unnecessary course for a music major), and found himself a slim, blue-eyed girlfriend. At the school year's end, however, when Mitch debonairly swooped into the pit and raised his baton to conduct "Bye Bye Birdie," my heart fluttered and I felt a pang of regret. He made a striking conductor with his curly black hair and lanky frame—the first student to ever be allowed to *conduct* the high school musical— and it didn't help that his twiggy girlfriend had nabbed the part of Rosie.

After my first year of college, my boyfriend and I broke up, Mitch and his girlfriend parted ways, and we serendipitously re-met in a hometown bar one summer night when he was off from Manhattan School of Music. We began "dating" (with Mitch this meant taking a walk in the woods or attending a Mahler concert with me driving since he didn't have a license). It turned out that, far from being a pothead, Mitch had never even tried pot, inhale or not. And he hardly drank, if ever (he was nursing a ginger ale on that particular evening). Two years after I graduated college, we became lab partners for life, mixing our chemistries to produce three remarkable, unique male offspring.

"That's the most awesome love story," Ben sighs.

I'm especially keen to recount it because of his dad's exemplary drug history. (I wonder if he notes I'm mum about mine.)

∞

Tonight at yoga, Tanya, the slim Asian beauty with serpent tattoos on her ankles, is subbing for Ali. As soon as we begin the opening poses, the cold that's been plaguing me all week slips away, just as when Mitch plays his clarinet in a performance, I never hear him cough, even when he's congested. He once played a holiday Pops concert with Skitch Henderson conducting while hiding a case of pneumonia; my stubborn husband didn't get to the doctor until he'd played the final note of "Have a Holly, Jolly Christmas."

Mind over matter, I guess, and I'm so happy to be moving and stretching after lazing about for three days. Only two of us are in the class tonight, and the woman next to me is an artist. I feel at home.

When I roll to my right side, as we do after Savasana, I open my eyes slightly. I notice a street lamp outside, trimmed with white holiday lights. I've been coming here since sunny June, but now it's pitch black outside, and rain pelts the windows. I experience a pure moment of complete peace; I love my family, my home, my life. I realize I haven't felt this content since before my mother died, but when I remember once again that she is gone forever, my contentment vanishes in an instant.

In that same moment, I notice the window hanging I've not paid attention to before: a copper butterfly. My mother and butterflies—how she loved them! At every birthday or holiday we gave her butterflies on soap dishes, towels, or candles; on every vacation, we sought out butterfly gifts to bring to her. My sister, my brother, and I, always searching for butterflies, even as adults, just as little children do when they learn that mommy likes a particular color, treat or flower.

Tears spring to my eyes as I gaze at the glistening streetlight, and I wonder how it is possible to be happy once again without her. It may be possible, in part, because that butterfly, that memory of my mother, is with me always.

∞

Snow flutters lightly through the sky as I head to class tonight, and I'm one of two students; a middle-aged man has come to class. He's a vocal fellow who sighs and groans through the poses as if he's having sex. I'm slightly embarrassed, but I won't let my inhibitions foil my practice. (I'd rather not have an unknown male nearby when I'm holding the Downward-Facing Dog pose for five long breaths—it's bad enough having proficient young women here when my ass is in the air and my nose near the ground!)

Ali is gentle, joining us in our asanas. I feel connected to her through the movements, more so than Jill, who is so far beyond me. Ali gives yoga as a gift, Jill as a challenge. I like both. Jill is clearly devoting her life to yoga; she isn't married, doesn't have kids, and loves to travel. The poses are her "work," and she doesn't go home to toddlers, teenagers, or a demanding husband. Ali, too. She's single, and a painter as well as a yogini. I wonder what I would have been like if I'd discovered yoga sooner. I wonder if I could have sent Aaron off to college without a tear, or said good-bye to my dying mother without nearly dying of grief myself. But I can't know, because there's no going back; I'm meeting yoga now, and we can only go forward.

Still, I feel envious of these young women. They have their whole lives to use their yoga, to make it work for them as wives, as mothers, and in their yogini-careers. Neither Jill nor Ali is a yoga dabbler—they're both as dedicated as nuns in an orphanage. When Jill leads us in three reps of "Om," her voice is clear and steady, filled with love and solid belief; when Ali bows and whispers "Namaste," you know that the divine in her heart is mingling with the divine in yours, even if you haven't really found your divine self yet. Yes, I admire and envy them, not just their heavenly bodies, but their sense of trust. I'd like to wake up each morning with the kind of trust in my heart that I can see in their eyes, knowing that however the day goes, it's the *right* way.

∞

Jill guides us in a silent meditation today. We're to repeat a mantra to ourselves, asking for everyone in the world to be happy. Dubious, I go along with it, thinking that me sitting in my yoga class wishing for happiness isn't going to change anything for the soldiers in Iraq or the people in the Sudan or those in cancer wards. Yet I suppose it can't make anyone *less* happy if I sit here wishing and hoping like a fool.

Across from me during practice is a thin woman who's been at yoga for ten years. I want to hurry up, to get to where she is, to get to where Jill and the others are who've been coming to yoga forever. But there's no rushing yoga. By definition, yoga takes time and patience. And more time. Standing still. And breathing.

I'm not going to make it to where they are by rushing and scrambling like a mountain goat. This is hard to accept because I yearn to discover why human beings have done yoga for thousands of years. And I want to know in a hurry: "Where's the fire?" I so often call to my kids as they rush out the door. Where, *indeed*, as Eloise likes to say.

But there *is* a fire inside me and I need to put it out; I'm in a rush to get to that calm and peaceful place inside that I can sense in Ali and in Jill. It's not that I want to *be* someone else; I just want to be the person I *am* without the baggage. I feel as if yoga is the golden ring, and if I don't grasp it soon, I'll never be able to find that peace I'm seeking. But of course, yoga is not so simple as that; and anyway, "grasping" is exactly what yoga is *not* about. I need to walk the fine line between reaching for yoga and letting it reach for me.

Christmas is almost here; it's always so sad now that my mother is gone, and yet I love the joyful underpinnings of the season. It's just that change thing again…it always creeps in during the holidays. Until a few years ago, after all, I spent every Christmas in upstate New York, in my parents' beautiful Victorian home (ramshackle as it was), with the formal dining room and fireplace (albeit a non-working fireplace), with my brother and eventually his wife and my nephew, and my sister and her kids and husband. My mother always served the same Christmas meal and treated us all as royalty—we *were* her royalty, her family. On Christmas night, Mom would sit in her pine green bathrobe, exhausted from the day's preparations, just drinking in our voices and faces.

So I try to recreate that now, and it's not easy. I shop and clean and make sure every person has a small pile of presents to open, and I cook my mother's exact dinner, even suffering over those idiotic baked beans she always made on Christmas Eve (though only Ruthann really likes them and she's not even here), which Mom must have baked for at least eight hours though until she died with her recipe undisclosed, I never paid any attention. I must have emailed or called my niece in North Carolina (sweet Lisa, the pastry chef) a hundred times this week, asking about those beans or the gravy or the pies. My sister and her family stay down south for the holidays now, but my brother comes to my house with his family, and Mitch's mom and sisters join us. His dear father died not long after mine, a few months after Sam was born.

My children expect everything to taste as it did when

Grandma was alive, and so I make the piecrusts from scratch and dash the cranberries with extra sweetening. I know my mother isn't watching. It's just that I want to keep her alive somehow, and maybe this is one of the ways. When I present Ben with a plate of sugar cookies just like my mom used to make, his face breaks into a relieved grin, as if he's been mourning the possibility that he would never see those cookies again. Well, cookies we can closely reproduce; not so Grandma herself, sadly.

I know I should be thinking of the "now," not dwelling in the past, but Christmas is inherently connected to tradition, and I'm not willing to relinquish my memories. This is part of my problem; I'm profoundly attached to the past. But I'd like to know who isn't! Jill, I'd guess. She seems to truly embrace the yogic concept of nonattachment. Of course, she doesn't have the motherhood card to play like I do…the card that trumps all.

Tomorrow is New Year's Eve, and today, in yoga, I'm noticing details about other women's bodies. I don't know why I'm focused on this, but for some reason I've decided I don't like the feet of the woman next to me; they're large and angry-looking, the feet of a stomping giant. As I ease into Warrior Two, I take note of the woman with a tiny star tattoo on her left shoulder. The tattoo works like an accent on her cream-colored skin, like a brooch strategically pinned on a jacket.

Jill squats next to me, demonstrating a pose. I'm amazed that her heels rest flat on the floor in a squatting position. She, too, has a tattoo—a glorious sunburst that spreads from her sacrum up her back. For the first time, I notice that Jill's roots are black. I'm surprised that she isn't a natural redhead. Somehow I think of Jill as having been born perfect—that's what she's always telling us, anyway. And if she was born perfect, why the need to dye her hair? Red does seem to fit her personality, though: vibrant, lively, and self-assured. As she passes near my mat, I see that she's not wearing toenail polish today. *Her* feet seem small and vulnerable without it.

Jill wishes us all a happy New Year as we leave, suggesting we enter the year with positive thoughts of something we hope to accomplish. I doubt that coming to yoga class twice a week for six more months is enough of a goal, but that's what comes to mind. I can't help worrying about what's in store; during this year, I'll have to find Sam a college. Aaron will graduate. Ben will turn fourteen. Sometime during the year to come, I'll have to face my children's futures. The thought of my boys being so young and so open to possibility, so uncertain, and so unformed, makes me see the need for my practice even more clearly. It's difficult for a mother to watch her child embrace the world, even if we want him to. But life is about change and growing and leaving, and I don't want to be standing in their way when I could be sending them off with joy and blessings. I wonder if it's possible for me *not* to become my mother, especially since I loved her so.

And I can't help wondering, too, if you've been loved as a child and you adore your parents (aside from a few adolescent years) whether that makes it harder than ever to blossom and survive in the harshness of the world. So many grow up with wretched childhoods. In a twisted way, I envy them; they have nothing to lose.

CHAPTER EIGHT: JANUARY

Upside Down

They say it's my birthday… January eleventh. Mitch and the kids bring home pizza and shower me with presents: loopy earrings, a necklace, a new purple nightgown— my favorite color. There's a carrot cake from the bakery and candles, but no one minds when I head off to yoga; the boys all have commitments, Mitch included.

I'm a good twenty years older than the other women who show up at yoga tonight, but I'm not thinking negatively of my age. I'm thinking, instead, of how lucky I am that my birthday falls on yoga night. I've been feeling the need to come to class strongly in the past few days. Memories of my mother, disappointing news about a wonderful administrator at my boys' high school, who the school board wants to fire, and world news—mudslides in the U.S. and the tsunami in Asia. The world seems like a terrible place, and yet, my own quiet existence— yoga, children, family—is a refuge. I suppose that's what family is for all of us, in its best sense, and it's why mothers in particular try so desperately to protect it.

I'm touched that Ali and the others sing happy birthday to me. They've found out from Natalie, who owns the center and keeps tabs. As they sing—Ali leading with a full, strong voice— I feel blessed. I'm a year older and half a year wiser, stronger, firmer, sounder, and calmer, I believe, because of yoga.

But I'm irritated when, at the end of class, some of the women immediately begin to chatter about the latest fad diet and where they're spending their winter vacation. I'm pleased that Ali suggests we put away our props—belts, bolsters and blocks—in silence. (And suspicious, yet again, of our teachers' phenomenal mind-reading abilities!) As we tiptoe across the room, placing these objects in the appropriate bins, I feel a sense of the silent magic of yoga.

"I wish you all courage for the New Year!" Ali calls out as we depart. And that really makes the class for me. Courage is a word I don't often hear on an average day, and certainly, not pertaining to anyone other than firefighters or cancer survivors. But every day does take some courage, and beginning a new year, after the one this country has just endured, we'll surely need it.

No sooner do I think I've made great progress, than I run into obstacles. Jill's class is unbearably tough, and I wonder if maybe growing a year older *has* affected my physical abilities. Of course I don't even attempt the ridiculous "Side Crow," apparently designed for women who weigh less than one hundred pounds and have been practicing yoga for twenty years. But even the more simple poses seem unreachable today, and I can't help noticing that the woman next to me—here for her second class—is attempting postures at which I'm failing.

Thou shalt not compare.

All this trembling and toppling must put me in a weakened state, for when I close my eyes in Savasana, I remember the last days of my mother's life, and realize that I was not nearly as attentive and kind to her as I should have been. I recall refusing to discuss what to do with her good china, even though the question was clearly troubling her. I sensed that she wanted to ask if I would be okay with it if she bequeathed the china to my niece, but I wouldn't give her the satisfaction of discussing the topic. It's not that I didn't want my niece to have the china; in fact, that's precisely what I wanted. I just didn't want to discuss anything to do with death, and certainly not with my mother. *She* was willing to face it, but *I* was not.

I was always so afraid of the topic that I actually banned the "D word" from my marriage ceremony. At my insistence, there was no "until death do us part" (but then, neither was there an "I do" from my nonconformist husband, who answered the preacher's "Do you take this woman…" with a simple "Yes").

Jill reminds us today, "Accept the things you cannot change," the yogic version of the serenity prayer. As tears slide from my eyes, I realize that memories fit that description: there is nothing I—nor anyone—can do to change the past. I can't erase the words I said to my mother and replace them with kind ones. I can't alter my memories, though I suppose I can select the ones I choose to dwell upon. I feel an overwhelming sense of sadness in yoga today, as if my failure to do the more difficult postures has led me to some of my other failures in life. But this is something we all must accept: there's no going back in time. All the more reason to live kindly in the present moment. I'm learning from yoga that the present moment is really all we have.

∞

El Presidente is inaugurated. I absolutely *flee* to yoga! How ironic that in the past year, our country has worked itself into a frenzied state of self-destruction just as I'm embarking on a restorative quest for inner peace. I wonder how I would be dealing right now with the war, the re-election of Bush, and the rebirth of intolerance in our country, if it weren't for yoga (and for Anneke, who's a rabid liberal and my political twin).

"I'm going to be teaching a hot yoga class on Friday mornings!" Jill announces. The power yoginis squeal with delight.

"There's no way I can tolerate any more heat than I am as a peri-menopausal woman," I retort.

Today, Jill asks us to be present in our movements. "Where are we? Here," she says. "What time is it? Now." I don't know if these are catchy phrases she's made up or if they're the hackneyed lines of ancient yoga masters, but I do know I'm always looking at my watch, planning what I'll do next. How liberating it must feel to be free of both the future and the past.

In Savasana, my stomach growls, and I remember that I'm meeting my friend Annie after class for brunch. (I assume Annie is a Republican because she's married to right-wing Billy the Vietnam vet, but she never shows her political cards.) A former school administrator, she's a wise and diplomatic woman with mischievous green eyes and a playful sense of humor— I'm really looking forward to seeing her. My thoughts wander over my plans for the day, and I feel a sense of anticipation; even though I'm supposed to be in the moment I find that today it feels good to look ahead. So often, in the past, I've awakened to days I didn't *want* to enter. Subway rides, lunching with a colleague for "business purposes," fears to be faced, ranging from driving a new route to conducting an interview with one intimidating expert or another.

I always work myself up into a frenzied nervous state before an interview, though once in conversation I'm lost in the joy of learning about a new subject or person. In fact, when I recall my very first experiences in the real world of journalism working for a weekly community newspaper, I'm surprised I garnered the guts to go down that road. My family—specifically, my dad— wasn't very supportive of my decision. When I drove away from home to live with Ruthann while I searched for a newspaper job and an apartment in the New Paltz area (I didn't have a trust fund to fall back on, or the means to backpack around Europe like many of my college cronies), I left my father (who wanted me to live at home and get a job as an English teacher) seething at the door. "You can't *do* this!" he cried out, as I threw my gear into my car.

But I painfully recalled my stint as a student teacher during the previous year at Kirkland. The memory wasn't pretty: I was so frightened to stand up before a class of fourteen-year-olds that I was sick to my stomach every morning and plagued by ghoulish nightmares. I remember once when one of the most popular, chatty girls in the class of tenth-graders confronted me during a vocabulary lesson as I explained that the word "boon" usually meant "blessing."

"What do you mean by *usually*, Miss Livingston?" she pressed, "Is there *another* meaning of the word boon?"

I realized that she'd caught me. "Umm, yeah, well it always means blessing. Unless we're talking about a *baboon*."

Obviously I wasn't meant to be a teacher, but at least the experience made me realize that teaching was my father's dream for me, not my own. This was a rare instance in which my fears actually helped me make the *right* decision, since I have no regrets that I've followed the writing path. But at first, my dad seemed to be correct: though I'd dropped my resume at every newspaper within a fifty-mile radius of New Paltz, all I could drum up was a waitressing job at a casual Italian restaurant. I certainly wasn't cut out for that either, and for weeks I woke in the night screaming,

"One large pie!" or "Small pie with sausages!" Never particularly graceful, I broke a lot of beer mugs, and once I unloaded an entire tray of a dozen sodas on a group of unsuspecting cub scouts and their parents. That was a seriously sticky situation.

One day in September after a busy summer of pizza pies, I heard back from a local newspaper. I drove my rusted blue Dodge Dart to the rather shabby basement office and met the editor—a thirty-ish man with a moustache and crooked smile. He handed me a piece of paper and pencil. "Make a list of all the ideas you can come up with for stories about a rocking chair."

"A *rocking* chair?" I repeated.

"I'll be back in ten minutes."

I began scribbling as fast as I could—who sat in it, who made it, the company that produced the wood, the little girl with the toothache whose grandma rocked her in the chair…the story of the pine forest where the wood was grown…

"If I don't snag this job," I thought to myself, "I'll be destined to dream either of cholesterol-laden pizzas or cruel adolescents forever! I *have* to get this job!" Who invented the concept of the rocking chair? Why is it comforting to children? What…

The editor stepped back into the office, carrying a cup of tea. He held out one hand and I deposited my assignment. I'd only come up with about twenty ideas, and I sat forlornly, eyeing the floor.

But then he chuckled. "I like these!" he smiled. "You have the job! When can you start?"

"Would yesterday do?"

I quit the restaurant and traded in my low-cut red blouse and short black skirt for a journalist's jeans and jacket. My job was to cover local politics and community news, and once a week to drive a delivery route—dropping off the very papers I had helped to write at little shops in the Hudson Valley. When I informed my dad that I'd nailed a writing job, he was jubilant, and immediately forgave my abandonment. He even presented me with a big container of dry, black cinders for my car, just in case I ever got stuck with my tires spinning in a snow bank on my route. "Never," my father warned, "ever, go anywhere on the East Coast in winter without cinders."

I was worried that I wouldn't excel as a reporter, but I had a sincere curiosity about others and I loved to write. My first assignment was to cover a school board meeting. As I sat in the audience furiously scribbling notes, I was horrified to find that the school board president was pointing a finger at *me*. "And *you!*" she bellowed, her voice shaking with anger, "What about that article your paper printed last week? It was totally out of line!"

This experience might have been enough to scare me off the track forever. But at just that moment, out of thin air, there appeared at my side a young man who had graduated from Hamilton a year ahead of me! We'd both worked on the *Spectator*, the college newspaper, and now he was in New Paltz covering the school board for a nearby city daily. He slipped into the seat next to mine and whispered in my ear, "Don't even respond. It's not your fault, and *she's* the one who's out of line!"

I followed his advice and continued to sit in a mute and frozen state. Sure enough, a moment later the board member moved on to another topic.

Eventually, I left that newspaper and got a position at a brand new start-up. The brilliant editor there called to offer me the job as the newspaper's very first reporter (he had once been employed at the other paper himself, and at *his* interview had come up with *one hundred* ideas to write about the rocking chair).

"If you want to be part of our staff you'll be at the Coach Diner at noon tomorrow for our organizational meeting," he said.

"Oh, I can't possibly do that. I'm on deadline and I'm due at the *News* at ten, and what excuse will I use to skip out in the middle of the morning?"

This editor had no patience for my whiney protests, and intoning some ominous carpe diem-style quote from Shakespeare that I can't now quite recall, he hung up.

I showed up at the meeting the next day, quit the other paper, and joined the fledgling *Huguenot Herald*, joyously working seventy-hour weeks until the venture got on its feet. This was a fantastic paper I was proud to be part of, and I realized in the year or so that I was there how vital it is to love what you're doing and do what you love.

CHAPTER NINE: FEBRUARY
The Yin & Yang of It

Tonight one of my classmates asks me how old my children are. When I recite their ages, she seems genuinely surprised. "You look *wonderful!*" she exclaims. Now, that's one of those backhanded compliments if I ever heard one. Do I look wonderful considering the fact that I've birthed three children who are now nearly grown, and for being my age (elderly)? Here I go again, with my negativity flowing. She talks about how hard it is to get to class with a baby at home. Yes, it's hard, even when the babies are grown.

I could have stayed home this evening; Anneke had popped in, and I wanted to chat with her about life and politics. It's difficult to get to the Center, to reach a narrow piece of mat where one expects heart, body and soul to change just a bit at a time. Half of the challenge is just showing up—being there instead of anywhere else, both physically and mentally. So often, in Savasana, my mind races, charging away from my body. I have to bring it back, calm it down, breathe and empty myself to become full. This is part of the allure of yoga; the slowness, the timing, the holding of the movements contrasted with the rushing whirlwind of thought. We are opposites; ha/tha, sun/moon, light/dark, life/death, male/female, yin/yang.

After class, I chat with Natalie for a moment; I'm beginning to feel that she's a friend, and I realize that I'm gradually gaining a sense of belonging. Sometimes, I'm still intimidated by the power yoginis, but more often I'm so soothed by yoga that I don't really care.

I say my good-byes and walk swiftly up our hill, ready for a cup of tea and bed. But as soon as I come into the hallway, Sam stops me in my tracks.

"The principal called," he says grimly. "I've been suspended from school!"

"What in the world…" my voice trails off, unable to fathom how this could be coming from the possible valedictorian.

It turns out that Sam's been nabbed for throwing a pen at another student (who has also been suspended for first jetting the pen at Sam). Stupid horseplay, but these days, schools are tough on kids; there's very little wiggle room in the disciplinary policies. Suspension is a serious issue at this point in Sam's life; he'll have to own up to this on his college applications, and knowing Sam, no matter how idiotic the reason for the suspension, he will never, ever lie about it on an application—or anywhere else.

My normally exuberant son sits on his bed like a deflated balloon caught in a treetop. He's no longer flying high.

∞

February is my least favorite month, and there's a scary young man at class today. Not that he appears to be an axe-murderer, but he has the look of a fit, experienced yogi and he's positioned his mat directly across from mine. Two minutes into our Sun Salutations, however, I hear Jill whisper, "Have you practiced yoga before?" He's a yogi virgin!

I think about how difficult my first time was. This guy seems willing to try most of the poses, but it must be hard to begin yoga in a room filled with women who've been practicing for months. I bet he's at least a little rattled by these powerful, shapely females. Of course, Jill is a very gentle teacher—even though she's demanding. If my first class had been with her instead of Ali, perhaps I wouldn't have started out with such an inferiority complex. I adore Ali, but I'll never forget how she refused to coddle me my first time out.

Even today, I'm wondering why it is that a woman at the other end of the room, who's only been coming to yoga for a couple of weeks, is able to get up into the Headstand. True, she has about one-fourth my body weight to haul upwards; she has the figure of a child. And she looks a good bit younger than I. Really, I don't know why I can't do an inversion. I know it's a little late in the game, but maybe I should just give this whole thing up.

As we rest, Jill's hands gently pass over me. "Quiet your thoughts," she chides softly. How can a woman who doesn't know my history, doesn't know what kind of tea I drink (or if I drink tea), doesn't know my kids, my husband, or my religion (or lack of religion), know me so well? And it's not just me; I notice Jill whispering to other students, and I see the gratitude in their eyes. (They may be dressed in stylish yoga clothes, but they can't really hide the fact that they're here for their hearts as well as their bodies.) She has some sort of sixth sense, or maybe it's just the gift of being "present." When you're near Jill, you know that she's with you; she is nowhere else.

When I arrive home, I'm still disgusted with my yogic ineptitude. Sam is in his room, reading a book. How silly to punish a kid like him, who so loves learning, for such a stupid kid-type thing as throwing a pen. Our whole system of punishments seems cock-eyed in this country. Either we're rewarding ourselves when we don't really deserve it or beating ourselves up for something that isn't our fault.

I race upstairs and shut the door to Aaron's bedroom (he's still away at college, and his is the only room with a bit of unused space in it). I don't know why, but after at least forty years of *not* standing on my head it's now at the top of my to-do list! I kneel and place my arms in Headstand prep, inches away from the door. What is the worst that can happen? I could crash and make a loud noise. I could put a hole through the wall. I could break my neck, and Sam would discover my body.

Here goes. I kick my feet up, one after the other, and lift with my arms pushing into the floor. Miraculously, my legs hit the wall and stay there. I am upside down! I am not falling! I'm still alive, and I am completely amazed. I haven't done a Headstand since sixth grade. I am fifty-two years old, standing on my head. Hallelujah!

If I can do it now, I can do it again. Just to prove it, I come down and then up a second and third time. Six months ago, this wouldn't have been remotely possible. Six months ago, I wouldn't have imagined this even in my wildest dreams! I'm laughing aloud like a crazy woman, and I don't even care.

I smoked a cigarette last night with Anneke, and this morning, as if to remind myself of this evil transgression, I begin coughing during yoga. I've brought along a water bottle, but I feel ashamed. Smoking is such an un-yogic thing to do. Yoga is all about the breath—honoring and revitalizing it—and smoking is the exact opposite. Many of my mortal habits seem so contrary to what yoga is about. It's not like the instructors are telling us don't smoke, don't drink, don't have a hamburger. But by coming to yoga, learning the poses, and listening to the respect the instructors have for the body and breath, one just naturally begins to want to clean up one's act. I wish yoga were a required class in high school; imagine how many kids could be saved from drinking, smoking, and drugs!

We have a vigorous class today, but I manage to keep up. I don't want to try the Backbend, though. It looks like a pose that should be reserved for people under forty, like those carnival rides for folks more than thirty-six inches tall. I'm waiting and thinking about the Headstand, and when Jill asks us to do our inversion, my legs simply float up to the wall, and my arms are strong, and I'm holding the pose.

Jill strides past me, turns and does a double take: "Look at this! When did this happen?" She can't hide her surprise! This feels like a rite of passage; the plump, middle-aged, newbie has made an important—albeit upside down—-step. Jill's teaching, my devotion, and the amazing capacity of the body to strengthen with time and effort have paid off. This must be nearly as gratifying for my teacher as it is for me (I imagine the power yoginis are thinking, "Lord! It's a miracle!") Jill is beaming as I look up and meet her gaze.

Before I leave the Center, Natalie calls me over to her desk. "I have to tell you something that may upset you. Ali's leaving. She gave me her notice and she won't be back."

"Not even to say good-bye?"

"She's already left. She took a job in the City and she started right away. I'm sorry. I'll miss her, too."

I can't hide my disappointment, but Natalie says brightly, "Not to worry, though! Tanya will take over the position."

To never see Ali again is a profound loss, but I remember Tanya as a teacher I could trust. I remind myself that life always serves up new teachers; there are always new people to learn from in yoga and everything else.

On my way home, I pass a new neighbor who's out working in her yard. She glances up from her task and cries in English with a heavy Korean accent, "You just keep looking younger and younger!"

"Thanks!" I smile. I know yoga is not really changing my age, but I do feel more vibrant as time goes on.

Once inside, I scramble up to Aaron's room, shut the door, and attempt a Handstand. I can't get up, not even close, and I fall to the side, my legs grazing the wall. I remind myself that just two weeks ago, the Headstand seemed impossible. If I manage to do a Handstand—and then, perhaps, Crow—I will really have made progress. I'll just keep trying; that's the best I can do.

As I sit cross-legged on the floor catching my breath, I realize that the only physical acts I ever saw my mom do were wringing laundry, swimming a sidestroke or juggling multiple frying pans in the kitchen. I'm asking my body, heart, and soul to do something that was never modeled for me (not that most mothers perform literal handstands for their children), but I *am* asking myself to go beyond what I've always thought of as my capabilities. In a way, I'm asking myself to fly when I was never given wings. And it's about time.

I missed class earlier in the week because of a virus, and now I feel weak and unsure of myself. As I place my mat down, the woman next to me sighs and comments that she also skipped class. "I hope I'll be able to get through this," she whispers. "If I can just get over that hump in the middle."

I'm flabbergasted by this confession; first, because this woman has been attending class for several years, and second, because she's actually spoken to me. Ever since my first day I've considered myself the "newcomer," the "outsider." Is it possible that others no longer view me as the incompetent yogini klutz? Even more surprising is learning that this woman—who appears so confident—still harbors doubts about her own ability to do yoga.

Jill takes her place on her mat, leads us in three strong reps of "Om" and then advises, "Try to speak kindly, and to have kind thoughts, and to do something every day that has a positive effect on others." Jill is a person who takes off her winter coat and gives it to a homeless woman, or who donates her favorite hiking boots to a poverty-stricken Mexican child. She lives her yoga in her actions, and she wants us to do the same.

As so often happens, I sense that Jill can see right into my soul –clear through to the more selfish, greedy aspects churning around in my center. Just this morning, I've gotten a call from Beth, my childhood friend, who lately seems only to phone when she needs a favor. She wants me to pick up her dry cleaning because she's home with a back ache, and even though I say yes, I'm thinking that I'll call her later and tell her that she can retrieve her own dry cleaning when she's better.

I've known Beth since I was five years old, and for decades we've been helping one another. (Strangely, we always end up living nearby; first in upstate New York, then in upper Manhattan, and now in New Jersey.) Lately, since Beth's divorce, it seems I do everything for Beth and she does very little for me. Each time she goes on vacation, she asks me to feed her menacing cat, an aggressive animal who bites and claws at my ankles ("affectionately" Beth claims) when I bend to place food in his dish. Often, while I'm in her empty apartment, I have a vision of a masked gunman swooping down on me just as I'm about to sprinkle Meow Mix into Arlo's bowl. Sometimes I imagine myself being wasted by the cat *himself* in some kind of clawing, Stephen Kingesque manner!

Hearing Jill's story, I realize I can pick up Beth's laundry. I don't know why it bothers me so much that the balance, at this time in our lives anyway, seems tipped. There's no need for equal portions of give and take between friends, and there's nothing wrong with being the one who gives (as long as I don't get scratched to death in the process!). Some day, the tables may be turned, and if and when that happens, I know Beth will be there for me. And even if the tables don't turn, I don't want to feel that I'm losing something by helping someone else. I glance around the room, and wonder how many other women are thinking that petite, sunny Jill holds a key to the deepest secrets within their hearts.

Jill says it's inversion time; from my upside down posture, I'm aware that the woman next to me isn't able to do her Headstand today. I can sense her astonishment when Jill walks by me and purrs, "Look at *you*, floating so nicely up there!"

I have no reason to gloat, but I do feel proud of myself. It may sound corny, but I feel as if I've made a new friend— my own body, my own self.

The month is nearly over; Ali is gone and we have Tanya to replace her. The class is all but empty—maybe some of the students have quit because they were partial to Ali. I miss her, too, but I won't stop coming to yoga because she's not here.

Tanya stands at the head of the class, a lean woman with a luminescent complexion and long, black hair in a braid. She speaks in a strong whisper. Her voice is kind, but hesitant, and I'm not flowing through the movements. I remember liking Tanya before, but now she seems somehow different. She's taken over Ali's class and she's going to make it her own; she even asks us to rearrange our mats. I'm lonely for Ali.

After yoga, I feel strangely unfulfilled, and when I sleep I dream that I'm in class again, and Tanya is chastising me for not taking yoga seriously enough. I wake up thinking that perhaps I'm taking yoga *too* seriously. I believe that's quite possible, even for the masters; in one book I've read that an ancient yoga practice involves sucking expelled semen back up into the penis. (I don't even want to imagine how that might work!) Reading about yoga, one learns many outlandish things; doing it American-style is, as they say, a whole 'nother ballgame. We Americans, of course, turn everything into marketing— colorful mats, T-shirts, tapes, charismatic gurus and seminars. I bet that willing one's expelled semen back to its origin would be a hard sell even in the U.S.A. I know my husband, for one, sure wouldn't buy it.

CHAPTER TEN: MARCH

Not a Competition

I spend the morning having a colonoscopy—just a routine check, now that I'm over the big 5-0, so I consider not showing up for yoga. But after enduring the procedure, my body is begging for restoration. Maybe I'm expecting too much of yoga tonight; perhaps I'd be better off with a nap.

Maybe I expect too much of yoga, period. I'm already wondering how it will help me get through my next ordeal as a mother. Sam is planning another airplane trip in May, this time to California to attend a prom and a reunion with friends he met at Oxford. And Mitch and Aaron are taking off for Japan (my husband is touring with the opera and has decided to bring our eldest son along as a college graduation gift). My family will be flying away from me, far from my grasp again. Only Ben will stay home; I have a few more years to harbor him. I was hoping yoga would, at some point, help me take flight myself. Still, I *do* feel a subtle shift in my attitude. At least I can now *think* about getting on an airplane without feeling faint.

At night, when I settle into my bed on my right side, I place my hands in prayer position under my cheek. I've noticed, the past few months, that this is the way I've been sleeping best. Each morning, I awaken the same way, with my hands gently pressed together. Before I began practicing yoga, I woke up each day with my hands clenched into tightly balled fists. I fear that this has gone on in my heart and soul as well.

∞

I can sense spring in the March air, and I'm thrilled to see that Jill is back from Mexico. Today she talks about being grateful, and I realize that's exactly how I've been feeling lately. As she speaks, a tear slowly winds down my cheek, rolling onto my lip; I taste its warm, salty flavor. It's fitting to experience the path of a single tear in yoga class, where we focus and concentrate, removing clutter and chatter from our minds. Normally when I cry—which I rarely *used* to do—my tears flow in generous cascades. But here in yoga class, the tear trickles down a narrow path, as if it's guiding me, urging me to pay attention to its source and destination. In this case, my tear isn't from sadness nor from joy, really. It's inspired by that sense of gratefulness that Jill is talking about, the realization that in a single day I have so much for which to be thankful.

I stare at my mat, noticing that the embossed lotus flowers on its surface are beginning to fade from use, and I'm rewarded by the knowledge that I've struggled and shown up enough to leave a physical mark. This is tangible proof not only of my efforts, but also of my constancy, for you don't wear something out unless you use it. The more my mat fades, the more I learn.

Jill is vibrant today, the room is full, and our mats are only inches away from one another. When we swan dive forward we must keep our arms in front instead of spreading them like wings at our sides. Though I prefer the intimacy of a smaller class, I have to admit there's something cool about twenty women reaching for the same poses. We're the yogini Rockettes!

"What would life be like without obstacles?" Jill asks. "Think how dull each day would be if we never had to face a challenge!" I admit I've never really thought of life in quite this way before, since I've always viewed obstacles as my enemies.

Jill lifts into a complex arm balancing pose, her legs in midair and out to the side. "Conquering obstacles," she smiles, "makes life exciting!"

I realize that I wake up most mornings hoping that nothing will send me off in an unexpected direction. When Sam twists his ankle in baseball practice or Ben calls and says he's gotten detention for some inane reason or Aaron breaks down on the highway in his car, I'm angry at the world. It doesn't seem fair that I have to contact road service for a kid who is "somewhere near a bridge on the New Jersey Turnpike," a kid who, after he calls me, locks his cell phone in the car. It doesn't seem fair that I have to race down to the baseball field and drag Sam to an orthopedist when I've just put a roast in the oven. Or fair that I have to call the principal and stick up for an honors student who's offended some little seventh grade girl by drawing a dopey face on a paper lunch bag and suggesting she wear it over her head. (But what *was* Ben thinking?)

I've never really considered these things—these obstacles— as gifts. Perhaps this is one of the stranger things about yoga; it opens the mind to simply looking at life from a different perspective. Maybe this is what comes of hanging with your head between your legs for so long or swinging your hips into Plow position.

When we "Om" at the end of class, the dissonant sounds of those who don't land on the same note please me. I have the most peculiar feeling…as if I'm becoming the woman I always wanted to be.

∞

It's St. Patrick's Day, and I wonder if the yoginis will be rushing home to boil corned beef and cabbage. (I suspect the hard-core followers will only be boiling cabbage, but my children would surely revolt if I stopped serving carnivore treats.) Today Jill advises, "Don't come to class with expectations. You'll be disappointed—don't arrive here thinking you're a failure if you can't do Headstands or Crows."

When Jill instructs us to go deep into a pose by wrapping our arms through our legs—a contortion I've never even attempted in the past—my arms just slide into place. I'm holding the pose before I even realize I'm in it, and I suspect that is one of the best ways to do yoga…to simply move into a posture without building it up in one's mind.

When I come home, I consider going upstairs to Aaron's room, against the closed door, and trying my Handstand, but no one's around, and if I kill myself my mangled body won't be discovered for hours. I don't know why I want to do a Handstand so much, but it seems that most of the women in the class have mastered it, and I want to be like them. This is my sickness, of course, and I need to get over it. I can imagine the yogini goddesses shaking their fingers, chiding me for wanting to master a pose just to keep up with the yogi Joneses. There are women in my yoga class who are twenty years younger than I, thirty pounds slimmer than I, with diamonds, manicures, pedicures, expensive yoga outfits, and exquisite cars. But it's not these things that I envy— it's their ability to place their hands firmly on their mats and kick into Handstand. Either way, I can see the yogini goddesses shaking their fingers: "This is not a competition." I *know*.

It's just that now that I know what yoga is, what it can do, how people who have practiced for years look and act, I want to be like them *now*. I'm as impatient as a kid who wants an ice cream cone on a sweltering summer night. But it doesn't matter what I want; there's just no getting there without putting in the time. The strange thing is, I *do* feel as if I'm on a timetable, as if there's some urgency involved in getting this right.

March is always blustery, and my van sways in the wind as I drive Sam to a nearby town for a haircut. He's talking about tricky ways to raise his GPA so that he'll be class valedictorian. He's neck in neck with a brilliant girl—they've been in an affable, academic competition since kindergarten.

"Forget about your GPA and just do the best you can," I tell Sam. "If you're valedictorian, great; if not, you know you're going to be salutatorian! Either way, you'll still be at the top of your class!"

"But I *want* this, Mom," he insists. "I want to be *first*."

I shake my head, "Just do your best. Anyway, if you start conniving ways to be first, it may simply backfire."

It's disturbing that my son is so hell bent on being number one. In my yoga state of mind it seems pointless, but then, I'm not sixteen years old. All his life, I've instilled in Sam a desire to excel. Now I wonder if we've gone too far, giving him the message that anything less than top gun is just not good enough. That's certainly not the lesson I want to impart.

Of course, I don't want him to give up his dreams, but I don't want him obsessing about ways to ace out a classmate either. In spite of the competitiveness that I sometimes feel in yoga class, I'm basically a person who'd rather sit back and let someone else win, because I do believe that winning is not always the happiest route. And yet I do want Sam—all my sons—to lead successful lives. It's just that the textbook definition of success doesn't always get it right.

∞

This morning, I ask Mitch to help me attempt a Handstand. He positions himself nearby, and I lock the front door. Don't want to take any chances on someone popping in and knocking me over. I peek out the window, too: I'm not keen on having the mailman witness my antics. But the street looks empty, so I place my hands on the floor, and kick up with all my might, pulling energy from my "core" as Jill has taught me. I soar up, my arms strong, my legs overhead.

"Way to go!" Mitch laughs. Gingerly, he holds my legs against the door, and then lets go of my ankles.   That's when I collapse in a crooked heap.

"Jeez, why don't you just lift weights?" Mitch cries, helping me up. He must think I've gone a little yoga crazy—and maybe I have.

Why *not* weights? I don't know the answer—other than the fact that weight lifting doesn't speak to my soul and makes me think of Hulk Hogan and Arnold Schwarzenegger, neither of whom I particularly want to emulate (though I loved the latter in "Kindergarten Cop"). But the deeper reason is twofold; first, I want to gain Jill's approval, and second, I want to prove that I'm not really my mother. The former reason is pretty stupid I'll admit, since Jill is so non-judgmental. Yet I can't help feeling that she's somehow disappointed in me, that I haven't lived up to her standards, and Handstand is part of this. Of course, I know that's my sick thinking again, but there it is. The second reason is more complex, because the Handstand is just a symbol, not a real measure of my similarity to my mom.

When I was a teenager I swore I'd never be like her; I saw a woman who lived and breathed family, who seemed to think only of what to serve for dinner and how to keep us safe. She had no outside interests, other than her church and volunteer work, and the way I saw it she had nothing to call her own. Even when I found her diaries after her death, they were filled with entries about trivial family matters—she wrote that my sister had chicken pox or that it was laundry day. But she never wrote about her *self*, about her feelings and hopes. She couldn't tap into that part of herself, except perhaps, when she was praying in the sanctuary on Sundays. (My mother didn't wear her religion on her sleeve—she simply lived it. Most of the religious people I know can come up with a lot of excuses for doing things they know Jesus really wouldn't approve of—but I never caught my mother making any excuses or doing anything that Jesus wouldn't think was just peachy.)

From the perspective of the Sixties, my mother was a failure –she was about as far from Gloria Steinem or Betty Friedan as a woman could get. So it was a shock, once I had children, to find how very much like my mother I'd become. Yes, I had my writing, and my career, but nothing was as important to me as my babies. Nothing is as important even now.

But if I could do a Handstand… I'll feel that I've crossed back over the bridge. Not that I *want* to be a ranting, bra-burning feminist any more (and God knows how I put up with not shaving my legs!), but I *do* want to reclaim some of the spirit and confidence of that time, a portion of that verve and courage I thought—as a teen—I would one day inherit (if not from my mom, from my generation). Avoiding being like my mother, I believed, was the answer, and when I failed at that, I sort of gave up. I didn't realize I could be like my mother and still push myself—that it was possible to be strong and independent and yet be motherly, soft and kind.

"Weights aren't my style," I answer my spouse. "So even if it kills me, I'm going to keep trying!"

CHAPTER ELEVEN: APRIL

Devotion in Motion

The chill is gone from the air, and when I step out to walk to yoga class, the evening feels light and warm. I hesitate at our door, listening to the clarinet notes wafting from the open window of our bedroom. I can also hear some crazy rock music—Red Hot Chili Peppers, I think the group is called—blasting from Ben's room. I remember my first days of yoga in the warm weather, nearly a year ago. For months now, we've been under gray skies.

In Savasana, I think of Ali, recalling the way she tiptoed around the room, stopping at each mat with her tiny vial of lavender oil, gently massaging our necks. She was the only teacher to regularly use the eye pillows— little bunny and whale-shaped creatures often used by the kids' classes. While missing her, I remember what Jill always says: "Everything changes." Two words that can bring such joy and such sorrow.

I need to accept what Tanya has to offer, and I think, in her heart, she just wants to teach us to be strong. I know I need to learn this lesson and perhaps my need is the very reason I resist. Like my mother, I don't want to push beyond my comfort zone—in yoga or anywhere else. Strength is something I've resisted; I've always chosen "I just can't do that" as the easiest route, but I should have learned from motherhood that "no can do" is not an acceptable answer. Motherhood requires strength, fortitude, and the ability to go not only above and beyond but higher and further—and I've proven in the past that I have the capacity to do so when it comes to raising my children. The question, then, is why do I deny this strength when it comes to raising up *myself?*

After class, I call upstairs to let the kids know I'm home. They're both on their computers, as per usual. Ben has told me he could not *live* without his computer. I find this hard to comprehend, since I spent my childhood soaking in the musty smell of maple leaves, the heat of the road outside my house, and the blue-red carcasses of worms on the sidewalk after rain. In my childhood, hollyhocks and bleeding hearts were magical, singsong phrases; mica in a rock garden counted as gold. A found orange salamander could be a beloved pet and I knew the smell of the lily of the valley at least as well as the aroma of Sunday's pot roast bubbling in Mom's Dutch oven.

Ben comes downstairs, blurry-eyed from too much screen time. He enters my little office where I'm now posted at my own computer, stopping to gaze at the needlework I have framed on the wall—a piece my mother used to keep in her hallway.

"Let me live in the house by the side of the road and be a friend to *the* man," Ben reads.

"It doesn't say *the* man, Ben. You know that."

"Yeah, Mom. It does. It says *the man.*"

"It means *mankind*, Ben."

Ben grins, grabs a water bottle from the frig, and shoots back upstairs to IM his friends.

The street we live on seems empty, as if no children inhabit our block. In fact, there are at least twenty, all in their houses, on their computers, or being carted back and forth to organized sports. The streets of the upstate New York town where Mitch and I grew up were teeming with children. Our shouts rang out in the thickening summer nights, and even as the sun went down we held claim to the street. In winter kids made snow angels and sculpted snowmen, working outside in the drifts until our fingers were frozen. I spent so many hours in the sun, snow and heat that my parents might have been conceiving babies inside unencumbered, for all I knew. We had tree houses and tree clubs, rules and regulations; we had muffins to bake from mud, stews to make of twigs and leaves. Outside was a world I knew intimately; the cracks on the sidewalks, the violets at the curb, the caterpillar eggs on the backs of the maple leaves—these were the markers of *my* childhood.

I bring Ben and Sam each bowls of strawberries; they glance up from their screens, delighted. I think of the teardrop-sized wild strawberries at the side of the road at the Adirondack lake where my family vacationed. They were so sweet, like deep pink sugar. I wonder if my boys will one day wax nostalgically about their mouse pads and the dusty taps of their keyboards. I wonder if they'll wish, as I often do, that childhood had never, ever ended.

Natalie opens our class today, reminding us that we're all part of the community of yoga. I admire Natalie—she's an astute entrepreneur, but she also approaches business with a yoga heart. She greets everyone as if we're part of her family, as if we're much more than just customers paying for physical and spiritual maintenance. Yes, I've come to feel that I'm part of this community, even though there's still a guarded sense of privacy among the members of the classes. We smile and trade pleasantries, but most of us are here for yoga, not for socializing.

I like this unspoken boundary; I'm reminded of the way I used to feel in church when the pastors started in with the practice of shaking hands with your neighbor or chatting with the person in the pew nearby. I was never comfortable, feeling that I'd come to talk to God, and if I wanted to shoot the breeze with one of the congregants it could very well wait until after the service. I suppose that's just one of the many things that turned me off to organized religion. And though yoga is not a religion, it sparks spiritual ponderings (especially when Jill is teaching).

Actually, Mitch and the kids seem rather surprised that I've stuck with a physical/spiritual pursuit. The Headstands and Tree poses in the hallway they've come to accept, but when I occasionally tell them about some of the spiritual topics we touch upon, they glance at each other with concern, as if they're afraid that Mommy may run off to an ashram in India and never come back.

I recall the one Easter Sunday when I seriously considered taking the kids to church; I'd located an ecumenical service at a local nature center. Mitch wasn't raised with formal religious instruction, and we'd simply taught the kids to be loving, tolerant, and to follow the *teachings* of Jesus. We'd read them Bible stories and insisted that they be kind to others and the earth (if not to each other!). Many of their religious friends, we noticed, liked to scare the crap out of our boys with predictions of how they were doomed to Hell because they didn't attend church. These kids would throw golf balls at passing cars or use racial slurs, and then go to confession to be forgiven. My boys were smart enough to see the lack of logic there.

Nevertheless, on this particular Sunday, I set the alarm, donned a dress, and proceeded to get the boys, who were then three, six, and eleven, ready to go. The Easter Bunny had made a stop at our house the night before, and the boys were up early anyway, noshing on jellybeans.

Suddenly, I heard a "whap" and then a squeal in the upstairs hallway, followed by another few "whaps" and more squeals. When I came to the top of the stairs I discovered they were having a fight using the colored hard-boiled eggs from their Easter baskets as ammunition; yolks and shells were caked on the walls and rug. Mitch, my dear husband, was still sleeping peacefully.

"This is a sign from God," I muttered to myself after screaming at the boys to behave. "These kids just aren't destined for formal religious instruction."

Besides, I'd gone to church every week my entire childhood and look where it got me. I always felt a lot closer to God when I watched a warbler darting from branch to branch in a tree than I did in a pew on Sunday.

I try to focus on class. I'm thinking of attempting a Handstand today, but when Jill tells us it's inversion time, I choose Headstand; I can get up so easily now. Since I started yoga at fifty-one, I calculate that if I keep practicing I'll look really "hot" by the time I'm seventy. Just in time to "meet my maker," as they say.

But if only I could master the Handstand, perhaps I can face Sam flying to San Diego, Ben going off to sleep-away camp, and Aaron and Mitch making their trip to Japan. I'm so afraid of losing the people I love—even for a week! Perhaps I harbor these fears for them because I don't want to face my own.

CHAPTER TWELVE: MAY

I've Gotta Crow

Aaron graduates from college today. We drive to his campus for the ceremony; the mid-May weather is perfect, and the college is in full bloom—not only the graduates, but also the cherry trees that line its walkways. Sitting in the stands at the huge outdoor stadium, I can hardly believe that four years have passed since we brought Aaron here, or that he's about to begin a new life. I remember being with my mother at his graduation from high school just months before she died. We had both fought back tears, one not wanting to upset the other. All our lives, we could just look into one another's eyes and know exactly what the other was thinking and feeling.

I know it's from my mother that I learned this profound fear of change, but again, it's from her that I learned to love so deeply. I remember how she used to calm me when I had a tantrum or a crying jag as a child, the same way she calmed this very grandson who's graduating from college today. She would take me (or any naughty or unruly child) into her arms and hug me; she would sing and rock and hold me close until the crying stopped. Never in my life did my mother raise her voice or fist— to me, or to any child. She certainly never called me a little fucker shit, or anything close!

I wish my mom were here now, not only to see how far Aaron has come, but also to witness how much *I* am changing. I wish we could share this moment of pride and happiness, and that she could know that my tears today are from joy. I squeeze Mitch's hand and smile at my mother-in-law, who's as proud of Aaron as we are.

And yet, it's a bittersweet experience, watching my first child meet life after college. I think back to that crazy, confused time in my own life—to the fight with my dad the day I left home, to my first newspaper job, to my courtship with Mitch, which was often rocky, and I pray that Aaron will have an easier time. I guess that's what all parents wish for their children, even though we know deep down that it's the *difficult* experiences that really help kids grow.

After the ceremony, I throw my arms around my son, and we smile for pictures, congratulations all around. But no one says what we're really thinking: "Welcome to adulthood, honey. Buckle on a seatbelt and brace yourself for a bumpy ride!"

It's nearly midnight, and Mitch is still at a gig. The kids—for once—have gone to bed early. But I'm waiting up, thinking about how differently I feel from a year ago when Sam was flying off to England. I'm not stoned on chardonnay, for one thing, and I haven't even felt the need to "tap." In the morning, Mitch and Aaron leave for Japan, and Sam flies to California.

Tonight at yoga, Tanya reminded us that one of the most important aspects of yoga is clearing our mind of chatter.

Throughout my practice I tried very hard to clear my thoughts, to breathe, to be in the present moment. I now have a set of skills that I didn't have before I began coming to the Center.

My friends have noticed that I'm calmer and so has Mitch. Even the kids seem to see a different mom. I do Tree pose in the upstairs hallway sometimes, and Ben laughs at me. He thinks I'm a little nuts, I guess, but I can tell he's enjoying the change. I don't chew my nails any more, or rant about politics as much. Maybe I'm just a bit kinder and more patient with others and myself. These are some of the things yoga has given me, but of course, there is much, much more. For the first time in my life I know that there's a fountain of peace inside myself—and it's not a mirage.

I hear Mitch's footsteps downstairs and when he comes into the room to change out of his tux, I greet him with a kiss and lingering hug. It was always hard when Mitch went on tour when we were younger, but now it's difficult in a different way. I'm not angry or resentful as I often was when the kids were little, and yet I feel a sense of yearning. For the first time in my life, I'm saddened not only because he's leaving, but because I'm staying home.

Mitch and Aaron are riding bullet trains and eating yakitori, but the daily drama goes on in our little town. Yesterday one of Sam's friends suffered a serious concussion after crashing into a brick wall while leaping for a ball during baseball practice. This makes me think about how the things that happen are often those we least expect. The obvious conclusion, then, is why do we spend so much time worrying? The bad will happen, just as will the good.

Yet for years I've done nothing but anticipate the bad moments, rehashing the gory details of every potential calamity in my mind, yet never being able to prepare for what really unfolded—my mother's diagnosis of amyloidosis, for instance, a rare and treacherous disease that I'd never heard of before the day a doctor at the hospital in Vermont revealed that my mother was soon to die from it.

Amyloidosis? Yes, in a way that was the Iceberg Theory in action—the unexpected, bizarre, untimely exit. And yet, the iceberg keeps on floating.

And even though Sam, Aaron, and Mitch have all taken flight, tonight I feel strangely peaceful. I'm looking forward to a quiet evening listening to the "ping" of Ben's computer and reading Jane Austen; I'm pretty sure I won't be having any panic attacks tonight.

Just Me and My Mountain

Jill is asking if anyone wants help getting up into a Handstand. If I don't do it now, I may never get up the courage. So I beckon her over.

"Should I give it a try?" I whisper timidly.

Her clear blue eyes light up. "*Of course!*"

I face the wall, bend over, and slowly position my hands firmly on my mat. Then, I kick my left foot up with all my power, lifting from my core. I soar up on the very first try! Granted, I only stay up for a fleeting few instants, and I can feel Jill's light touch on my ankles, but nevertheless, I'm up there, and I don't topple over or break my neck. Jill bends and puts her face close to mine.

"How do you feel?" she asks.

"I feel damn good!" I gasp. A miraculous flow of strength

and energy is coursing through my body. I'm the indomitable queen of an upside down world! I wish I could do Handstands all day long!

My classmates are clapping and cheering—even the power yoginis. Everyone knows how hard I've worked to get here, but I'll bet only Jill truly believed I ever would.

∞

My anniversary is here; one whole year of yoga, twice a week, every week! I'm amazed that I've stuck with yoga this long, and even more amazed that I've given up all intention of ever quitting. Here I am, at the end of a year, and when I look back I see a very different woman.

I still fear losing my children—to growing up, to college and beyond. And I still miss my mother every day. But when I think of how much worse this fear and loss would feel without yoga, I'm so grateful. Yoga has given me a quiet space in my mind where my sorrow and worry simply can't enter. Before yoga, I simply could not find that space, didn't even know it existed.

Our session is challenging and there are new members who can bend and fold like human pretzels; I do envy them, but I no longer think only about how plump and clumsy I am. Instead, I'm thinking about how I can keep reaching and trying, and about the day when I'll be able to do that damned toehold and stretch my leg out straight while balancing on my other foot. I believe that day will come, and who knows what kind of thoughts and spaces in my mind will open when it does.

I manage another Handstand today, with Jill's help. I should be jubilant, but I'm rather disappointed because my arms shake and I can only hold the pose for five seconds. While I'm up there, though, I notice another woman in the class smiling at me, as if she's proud. She's watched my progress this year, and even upside down, I can tell from her joyous expression that she knows how far I've come, and that she's happy for me.

It's funny, because I remember feeling happy for *her* when she first did a Handstand, and I realize that, though we don't really know each other well—just first names, some of us—we're pleased for the others in our classes, as we watch each other stretch and grow into better yogis and better people. It *is* a community, and even though most of my progress and change has come from within, I also feel that I'm part of something larger, a uniting of individuals who really *do* desire not only strong and beautiful bodies, but also peaceful hearts.

I bend into Child's pose and take five deep breaths.

Today, as if she knows I've been coming to yoga for exactly one year, trying to figure out what it's all about, Jill opens the class by asking, "Why do we come to yoga? We are here to forget. We come to forget the chatter in our minds, and the doubts and fears and worries, and to put everything aside and go to a quiet place. And…we come to remember; to remember that we are perfect, that we are born perfect, without flaws and self-doubts."

She sums it up nicely, precisely what I've been trying to figure out this past year. Of course, I do know we come to forget—at least, that's the outcome. But it's not as if I purposely slip into my yoga capris and camisole and run out to escape the dirty dishes, and my children's problems, and the memory of my mother's death, and all my troubles. But that's what happens, if only for an hour. So she's right about that; yoga is a clear way out of the mind's jungle.

During our practice, we arrive at a quiet, resting Child's pose, and as I close my eyes, I think fondly of Aaron; he's home from college now, but one day he'll be moving to his own apartment. He's interviewing for jobs, and when I see him dressed in a suit, driving down our street in his car, I can only imagine that before I know it he'll be getting married, and having children, and building a life of his own. Change: the thing I fear so much.

But yoga is not just about forgetting and remembering; it's also about dealing with loss and leaving. My whole life, it seems, has been a series of arrivals and departures. All our lives, in fact. Until this year, I didn't handle these things very well; the thought of any of my children growing up and going away, boarding airplanes, going off to college or moving, all seemed unfathomable, and so painful. My mother's death was something I couldn't emotionally touch before yoga; the change that her absence brought has been greater than I ever could have imagined. She was my best friend; in my heart, she still is.

When I think of what my yoga teachers have imparted this year, and especially Jill and Ali, I realize that they've helped me— and the poses have helped me— to somehow accept (I'd like to say embrace, but I'm not quite there yet) change. Maybe it's something to do with the movements: the Cat and then the Cow, the twist to the left and then to the right, the reaching up, and then bending to the ground, the constant training of the body to move one way, and then to move in the opposite way. Hatha: sun, moon opposites, dark and light, yin and yang. This must be key in the way yoga shapes the mind and heart, in the way it helps one to understand that every movement has a counter movement, that every action has an opposing action, that the happy parts of life will be met by the sad, and the sad, in turn will be met by the happy.

In the past, I was always running or hiding from the sadness: death, loss, leaving, darkness, change. I was so afraid of all these things that I feared them more than I valued life, giving, receiving, light. I was guided by fear, and most of my decisions—to write or to teach, to take certain assignments or not, to travel, to step anywhere outside the zone of familiarity and comfort—were the byproducts of my belief that "No, I can not do that"—*whatever* that was. But I now see the glimmer of possibility that one day *I* will be at the front of the line, that one day I won't be guided by fear and self-doubt, but by the strength within my own heart.

Yes, I know I have much to learn, but if one year of yoga is any indication, I look forward to what I might come to understand in the future. I'd love to find a firm surface where I can stand in Tadasana—finding my "mountain," a place where I am grounded and confident even while life swirls with change around me.

"Let's do Tree pose!" Jill suggests. "We'll hold twenty breaths on each foot."

We ease into our positions, our arms outstretched to the sky like branches, one knee bent as we balance. Jill counts aloud. Some of us topple over after five seconds, some last fifteen, and some of us—myself included—stand still and strong up to the close of forty breaths.

I want to be standing tall, my hands in prayer position, unafraid and holding my own in my life, and after this first year of yoga, I actually feel I am on my way.

In the back of my mind, however, is that niggling little Iceberg Theory. It's often when things seem most right with the world that the ice can begin to crack.

YEAR TWO

*"Anything 'bad' that happens in your life—
use it for enlightenment."*
—Eckhart Tolle

CHAPTER FOURTEEN: JULY
Child's Pose

Yes, I'm in my second year of yoga; I'm on my way—but to where? Mitch says I'm turning into a yoga junkie, and he can't understand why I need to attend class to practice. He also suggests that yoga is something that bored, affluent housewives do, like fondue parties in the Seventies (which recently have come into vogue again, I've noticed). I can't believe that yoga is just a fad for these women, and it seems blasphemous to compare this ancient practice to dipping bread in hot cheese (or even strawberries in hot chocolate!).

Anyway, I'm not affluent by a long shot. I'm certainly not bored either, though summer has made me lazy. Tanya is leaving for Spain this week, and I have to admit, I need a break from her rigorous classes (the yogini teachers certainly seem to have wanderlust!). I still miss Ali; I'd like to run into her some day, just walking down a street in Manhattan.

After class today we visit Columbia University; time to start looking at colleges in earnest for Sam, as much as I hate to admit it. Standing in the June Manhattan mugginess, a Columbia brochure perched on my head to protect from the sun during our tour, I think of Gino, Sam's best friend, who was diagnosed with cancer this year. I wonder if Gino will be filling out college applications in the fall, whether missing half of his junior year will affect his chances of admission to a good college. We've known Gino since kindergarten—a bright, sweet-natured kid originally from Italy. It suddenly seems so silly, fretting over whether Sam will get into an Ivy League when Gino's parents are probably wondering if their son will be going to college *anywhere*. I feel sick to my stomach whenever I think of what Gino's family must be going through, and when I glance at Sam, I'm overcome by the realization that, rather than the opposite, a mother's life is really in her *children's* hands.

Everything seems different now that summer is here. The kids stay up late and sleep all morning. Aaron is living at home again, which is odd. I guess I thought after college he'd never return. I was so afraid to have him leave and admit that our family was changing, and now he's back again, which requires even more changes. He's still looking for a job, and not having much luck. I remember my summer back home after I graduated from college and how miserable I was to be living with my parents again, as much as I loved them. By September I'd found my own apartment in New Paltz, and not long after, my newspaper job. During that heady year of freedom, Mitch and I stopped dating for a while. I needed to sew some wild oats, and New Paltz was a great place to do it— a bustling college town nestled in the scenic Shawangunk Mountains. Mitch wasn't too happy about that; he would have preferred to marry right away, but I just wasn't ready.

One night, after a heated argument on the phone, I told him I was taking the bus down to the City so we could talk in person. "I'll get in around 1 a.m., so you'd better be there to meet me," I instructed.

When I arrived at Port Authority, Mitch was nowhere to be found. Manhattan's lively bus station was not exactly a chic place to linger in the middle of the night, and as I waited, shifting seats in the lobby to avoid the muggers and drunks, I became increasingly infuriated. How could he leave me sitting there at three in the morning? An hour later, I boarded the next bus out of Manhattan, crying and cursing all the way back to the bucolic countryside.

Later that morning I called my nasty boyfriend. "I never want to see you again!" I snapped.

And thus my wild-oats sewing began, a wonderful time, from my perspective. I was a free woman who answered to no one other than my newspaper editor; I had an active social life, my own car (unreliable as it was), and my own cozy studio apartment. I loved driving through the fog and falling leaves on an autumn morning, and my job at the *Herald* rocked.

But one night after covering a late town planning board meeting, trundling home in the snow, I realized that I really didn't want to live this way forever. I wanted to be with a man I deeply respected and loved, and one day, maybe, have a family. There were plenty of interesting male prospects to choose from in those days, but only one I knew who really fit into my vision of the future. My piano teacher—a bit of a clairvoyant—had always told me to envision exactly what I wanted in life and it would come to me. Whenever I closed my eyes and thought about my romantic future, I'd always see the same weird things: a music stand, a metronome and a purple Victorian couch with white lace antimacassars. I figured this either meant I was destined to marry a musician or I was going to be a museum security guard.

One evening in the summer, nearly a year after Mitch and I had parted ways, I came home to find my phone ringing. "You seem to have left your nightgown in my apartment," Mitch said. "I'd like to return it to you."

"Oh, yeah?" I remembered that nightgown— an ethereal ice blue swatch of cotton.

"And I still love you."

"Well, I still love *you*."

The following June, we married.

The Fourth of July holiday weekend is here, and on Saturday morning, we tool through Brooklyn, en route to dropping Sam off at Pratt Institute to attend three weeks at a summer pre-college course, which seems to be all the rage lately. We pass a number of attractive brownstones before pulling into the campus lot.

By the looks of the quad (freckled with lots of kids with green or purple hair and nose rings), Pratt will be an education— if not in architecture (which is what Sam wants to study), at least in how an artsy-fartsy school (as we used to call them) works. I went to such a school myself—with lots of pottery and dance majors. Of course, just across the street from Kirkland was our venerable coordinate institution, Hamilton College, and one could take a proper, traditional philosophy or science class there, or opt for a Kirkland class, where students called the profs by their first names and sat on the floor smoking cigarettes with dogs sprawled at their feet.

But our son is hoping to get into Princeton…. rowing, fencing, supper clubs.

Sam unloads his gear and nonchalantly bids us adieu; after all, he's a world traveler now. "I'll call you if I need anything," he quips as I hug him good-bye.

"You'll call us even if you *don't* need anything," I scold. We watch him disappear into his dorm, and then head back to New Jersey.

∽

I awaken to a sweltering mid-July day, but in spite of the rising temperature, I make the mistake of attending the Power Yoga class. I've been at yoga for a year and I will not be intimidated. Jill is teaching, and it's the only class I can fit in this week.

But the class is far above my level, and half way through I get stomach cramps. Maybe it's some kind of peri-menopausal glitch. Or maybe I'm getting sick. Or maybe I'm just….too old for this.

I slip into Child's pose, furtively checking my watch, and opt out of the inversions, trying to become invisible. But one can't hide from Jill; her comforting hands caress my shoulders, telling me without words that it's okay.

In the afternoon, we visit Sam at Pratt. He's glassy-eyed and silent and I don't know what's happened to the exuberant child-teen we dropped here a week ago.

"It's the junk food I've been eating," he says, "plus the lack of sleep, and the ridiculous amount of work they throw at the architecture students."

"Are you sure you want to pursue this subject?" I press. I'm beginning to hear that everywhere the architecture and engineering students struggle harder than anyone on campus. I don't really want my son to get into a college where they pummel the students to death.

"I *think* so."

"Maybe you should switch your major to English," I suggest. "All *I* did in college was read books, write papers, bullshit about the books, and party."

Sam brightens. "*I* like to read," he says.

CHAPTER FIFTEEN: AUGUST

The Art of Acceptance

I'm glued to my computer, ruminating about what to do about Sam and his suspension question. I search online, and find a site that discusses the problem. Naturally, all the college admissions officers advise kids and their parents to tell the truth. Taking responsibility for your actions is what counts, they claim. Still, it's clear as day that if two kids were neck and neck for an Ivy admission, the one with a suspension would get the rejection.

While I sit here worrying, Sam is out at Gino's house—the boy with cancer who has missed four months of school, who didn't get his license this year, or attend the National Honor Society inductions. Right now getting into an Ivy is about as far from Sam's mind as it can be. He's more interested in having fun, being with Gino again, reconnecting with the girls from town he lost pace with while he was at Pratt. He seems content, in fact, with the idea of applying to schools that aren't so competitive. Maybe this college quest for an Ivy is *my* problem.

Yoga has taught me that life is not about competition, but it's hard not to fall into the trap, especially when we want what's best for our kids. Still, I know that I must accept whatever happens; and whatever happens will be right for Sam. It's rare to find such a motivated student; I remember the five-foot Native American totem pole he made in seventh grade from cylinders, paint and feathers. And then there was the suit of armor he constructed for a friend, and the complex woodland miniature. I should have known he'd want to be something like an architect, even then. It's weird the way life tells us what to do, even when we're not paying attention.

I glance at his picture above my desk, right next to a cute little note he penned when he was in grade school that I've taped to my wall. "Thank you, Mom," it says, "for giving me all the love you could." I always wonder if he meant I didn't give him *enough* love; it nearly sounds as if he's forgiving me for not quite living up to his standards. But I can't imagine loving my kids any more than I do. I guess he just meant, "Thanks for the love, Mom."

I can't control the college outcome, so I might as well take a more yogic attitude of acceptance. We need to accept ourselves, our teachers, our classmates, our lives and abilities. Some might think this sounds a bit like a religion, but that's not it. I don't really care if anyone else shows up for class, and I'm certainly not planning to go door to door distributing the yoga sutras. Though it might be sort of fun, next time the Jehovahs stop by, to have a copy on hand!

We're back on the Cape for our yearly visit. We hike, swim in the kettle pond near the cabin, and Eloise and I spend the evenings watching the sunsets and talking. We like to sit outside on the deck after dinner with our cups of coffee or glasses of wine. The boys are inside, playing music or using the computer.

Mitch listens while Jeb practices the bassoon, and several times during our visit they entertain us with duets. But for Eloise and me, the best part of our visit is just talking, so we often stroll down to the pond together or make up excuses to drive to the store. ("We can't possibly serve dinner without fresh parmesan!") Marriage, motherhood, kids, books, our hopes and disappointments, we talk about everything that matters to us. We make each other laugh, and there are no uncomfortable silences—only the silences that we choose. Of course, we also hit the beach for yoga.

In the past, Mitch may have been a bit envious of my friendship with Eloise, but he's come to love her dearly, even though they've had their quarrels. Once, Eloise sat Mitch down and had a "talking to." For years, Mitch detested holidays and celebrations of all sorts; Christmas, Valentine's, my birthday. The only one he would acknowledge was our anniversary, which he said each year was a true accomplishment (I *am* aware that marriage to me is not always a picnic). But the other days would go by without a card or present, and sometimes with a nasty commentary about the waste of money they entailed for the poor suckers who observed them. I'd always complain to Eloise, until one year she'd had enough.

"I understand that these holidays mean nothing to you, and that you'd rather not acknowledge them, but they're not about *you*, they're about your wife, and she enjoys celebrating. So from now on, you need to buy her *something*," Eloise lectured my spouse.

"But it's all so stupid," Mitch replied.

Eloise shook her head. "It doesn't have to be expensive, just a little gift or card, because it will make *her* happy."

And so surprisingly, from that day onward, that's exactly what he did.

I love the fact that Mitch listens to Eloise, because he

listens to very few people. But he and Eloise really have a lot in common; they're both people who look you in the eye, to whom waitresses tell their life stories, to whom shopkeepers divulge their secrets, who can go just about anywhere and speak to anyone and come home with an intimate, personal tale, freely offered up by whoever they've encountered. I find it curious that two people I love so much are so alike (and yet so very different). They share a certain kind of wisdom and openness of heart.

After Eloise's annual special seafood dinner of scallops sautéed in butter and garlic, lobster tails, shrimp, and clams on the half shell, her hubby takes our kids and their dog for a walk, Mitch loads the dishwasher and Eloise scours the last of the pots and pans while I do the sweeping and straightening. Sometimes, I wish I could be married to them both. Certainly, Eloise is the better cook. But Mitch makes a mean decaf cappuccino.

August is half over; I'm back in Jill's class, and I feel as if I've gained about ten pounds while on vacation. I can hardly lift my butt into Downward Dog, but I concentrate on my breath, and I manage to keep up with her "flow." I think about the fifteen-mile bike ride I took on the Cape and how I woke up the next morning with a horrible charley horse in my calf. Mitch had said, "There, this proves it. Yoga is for wusses." Of course I know this isn't true, even if my biking legs are already in retirement.

I've read in a magazine that people are practicing yoga *in the nude*. This is something I don't even want to think about, let alone visualize. If Jill ever suggests we fling off our clothes, I'm outta here.

After class, I come home to trip over a huge pile of envelopes in my doorway. As the school year approaches, the mail is flooded with college brochures and applications.

I place the latest brochures next to the toppling mound on

our dining room table—it's already a foot or more high, though Sam is only applying to eight schools (I've heard tell of kids who apply to more than twenty). The U Penn application alone is thirty pages long. Each time I walk through the dining area I glance at the pile, thinking about how it will destroy my autumn strolls in the morning sunlight, my newspaper deadlines, and even my calm relationship with my middle son. I can't imagine how Sam and I will get through this process without at least a hundred disagreements.

This would be a good week to get moving on that pile, since Ben is away at a computer camp. (I know he's on the computer too much as it is, but it's vacation and we thought we'd humor him.) Plus, the house is doubly quiet now that Aaron has found a computer job in the City. He'll live at home until he saves up enough for his own place, which is fine with me. I know some parents are in a hurry to boot their older children out, but sometimes kids of all ages just need a nurturing place to land. I've inherited my mother's ability to gather and nourish—but I also wish I'd learned more about accepting the ebb and flow of life.

I walk swiftly to class today. Jill is back, glowing and energetic after a trip to Baja, where she attended some kind of weeklong yoga marathon. The yoga teachers sure know how to enjoy life; not only do they spend time practicing, meditating, and eating healthy foods, they also get to traipse off to fancy spas all over the world to study with master yogis and refine their asanas. If I had a few yoga buddies and some extra cash, I'd be tempted to steal away to one of these places myself. But then there's that small matter of the airplane— I rather doubt anyone would want to *drive* to Baja with me.

Today Jill talks about looking at life with a positive attitude; she says that we shouldn't always wake up in the morning and whine, "Oh, it's a rainy day!" Instead, we should try, "Rain! Just what the garden needs. I won't have to water tonight."

"On my retreat," Jill recounts, "I was awakened each morning at the crack of dawn by a rooster! Instead of cursing the bird, which was my first impulse, I learned to welcome his early morning cry to start my day. Why be mad at a rooster, who's just doing what he does? He made a great alarm clock—even though I couldn't control him!"

I abhor this Polly-yoga mentality, but I have to admit it's true. Too often I wake up in the morning dreading the day. Jill actually believes that we can make our own day by thinking about it in a positive way. My method is to just avoid doing things I don't like.

Tonight I surf online, searching the college websites for gritty details. I've forgotten about the interviews required for architecture students and now I begin to obsess about when we will fit these in. I don't worry about how Sam will do at the interviews or what he will say; he's an amiable kid so I leave such matters up to the gods. But I'm mighty fearful that I—the Mom—will screw up the timetable. There seem to be more details and demands in this line of work than when I was managing editor of the photo magazine.

Mitch, always the sage, stops at my office door on his way to the kitchen for his customary evening cup of tea. He's grateful that I'm handling this college project (he's more allergic to the computer than I am to caffeine) but he also sees I'm taking it to extremes. Of course, he's already worrying about the finances—college these days costs as much as a house.

"Don't make too much of this," he reminds me. "Sam will be fine wherever he goes."

CHAPTER SIXTEEN

September: Water, Water Everywhere

It's September and it still feels like pool weather. Unfortunately, the weather hasn't been so kind to New Orleans, where Hurricane Katrina has caused massive destruction. In yoga, we dedicate our practice to the victims. Lives can be swept away in a heartbeat, and this makes everything—even yoga—seem inconsequential.

A hurricane is the perfect metaphor for so many things in life; how swiftly everything can vanish, in a nanosecond. The good thing about yoga is that it reminds us that things can also turn the other way. We have to believe that just as darkness falls every night, so will the light return. No "Iceberg Theories" for Jill; she has a positive spin for everything.

Jill catches me off-guard today. "Have you done your assignment?" she asks after we "Om." I stare at her blankly, wondering if I was supposed to be balancing on my nose over the weekend.

"I asked you all to write down your first thoughts when you woke up!" she chides. Indeed, some of the yogini ladies are revealing theirs: "I need to walk the dog!" or "Wow, what a gorgeous morning!"

I've forgotten, and I'm somewhat embarrassed. I promise myself I'll pay more attention next time; my mind seems to be wandering lately. Back to school, a change in schedule, financial concerns, and of course, Katrina.

On my walk home, however, it comes back to me. My first thought this morning was just: "Should I get up or go back to sleep?" Not very profound, yet I realize there may be a deeper message. Since the town pool closed on Labor Day, I've been so morbidly tired that I'm taking a nap every day. When I wake up, I'm irritated with myself. I'm not writing, drumming up assignments, trying to make money to help support my family; no, I'm sleeping in the afternoon like some sort of slug. So the question of whether to get up or go back to sleep goes a bit deeper: Why do I want to avoid the day? I'm listless about life in general lately, and I don't know whether it's just about Sam leaving, or if it's something more.

The shoes are already filling the cubbies when I get to class today. After a year of yoga, I do wonder why it doesn't really seem much easier. Yes, I can get into a Headstand, and I can do the Plow, but my bones still creak and sometimes my legs feel heavy and unbalanced. The simple fact is: yoga is not easy. And it doesn't get any easier as time goes by. That's probably why women who have been practicing for years and I can both enjoy the same class. Even though we're at different levels, we're all pushing ourselves.

I manage that damned yogic toehold today for an instant, but then fall over. Jill says, "Great!" when she sees me trying, and I feel like a kid in grade school again. At the age of fifty-two, I'm excited that I can almost stand up straight while holding my toe and stretching my leg out. But it's nice to worry about what the body can and can't do for a change. I'm tired of worrying about the Katrina victims, the incompetence of Bush, and where Sam will get into college. It's comforting to just think about holding onto my big toe.

After class, I leaf through Sam's U Penn application. The number of pages and essays bewilders me, as does the fact that the forms are numerically arranged, and yet have other forms plunked into the middle with a line that reads "please do not separate these pages." I rest my head in my hands in frustration. If I were a high school student I'd chuck this application in the garbage, go back to smoking pot and having sex and settle with a community college. I don't know when teenagers even find time to have sex these days!

I turn from the college pile, devoting the rest of my afternoon to a newspaper article. But during dinner, I can't resist warning Sam about the application; it won't hurt to prepare him for what lies ahead.

"The U Penn application has really weird pagination and instructions," I comment.

Sam regards me quizzically. "All that means, Mom, is don't separate the pages within a single form from *one another.*"

I know that Sam is smarter than I, but isn't it unnatural when a kid can follow directions better than his mother? It sort of disrupts the cosmic order, and when I tell him to go to bed tonight, I almost wonder if *he* should be turning off *my* light.

∽

I sit at my computer today, looking out the window at the end of summer impatiens in their pots on my deck, their pink and white flowers perched on long stems. I'm so grateful that certain flowers last all summer and that others—like the mums—are just opening their buds to autumn. Jill talks about this all the time, telling us that we should focus on generosity and gratefulness, two qualities that really enrich life.

More than Jill's Handstand, I envy her attitude. I wish I could have even an ounce of her optimism. Whenever I ask Jill how she is, her answer is always, "Great!" The funny thing is, I think she actually does feel great most of the time. I believe it's because she's focusing on the aspects of life that offer beauty and hope; she doesn't let her mind travel down the roads that my mine frequents. It's as if her thoughts are habitually sitting at an outdoor café in the Paris sunshine, while mine (if my thoughts would fly) are lurking in the dark alleyways behind the garbage cans. But it also sort of feels like Jill has gotten up from the table, noticed me, and gone chasing into the alleyway with a big stick. "Get out of there!" she cries, rattling the cans. "Sit down over here by me and breathe!"

In the afternoon, Mitch and I walk to the nearby high school where we're to meet Sam and the guidance counselors to discuss that little suspension question, which has now popped up on five of our eight applications. One—a tall, lanky woman whose own kids attend a pricey private school— suggests that we simply lie; Sam didn't really deserve a suspension, anyway. "Just leave it off the application!" she suggests, "otherwise it'll come back to bite you!"

The other counselor looks Sam squarely in the eye. "I'd like to advise you to lie, but I can tell that your heart is torn. It just doesn't seem to be something you'd be comfortable doing."

And neither would I: I can imagine Sam at his graduation from Princeton— magna cum laude of course —but just as he steps up to receive his diploma, an elaborately decorated dean with golden cords flying from his robe races down the aisle, frantically waving a paper above his head. "Halt!" he cries out, "This boy can't receive a diploma! He lied on his application! We've just learned that when he was seventeen he was suspended for violently hurling a Bic!"

Anyway, the kid just isn't a liar...if he was, he'd have fibbed his way out of that ridiculous suspension in the first place. We leave the meeting with the sense that nothing has been accomplished, though one of the counselors has volunteered to look more deeply into the matter and let us know her findings.

Back at home, I can't shake off a deep sense of gloom. I pick up that U Penn application again and scrutinize it. Sam spends the evening watching football and hanging out with Gino, who is miraculously on the road to recovery and hoping to attend Rutgers next year. I realize that if we don't get moving, Sam will never fit in all these interviews and be able to get a portfolio together. Finally, he pens a paragraph about the activity that most interests him, but the writing seems uninspired, and the fact that he's been in band since seventh grade no big whoop. He didn't conduct the all-state choir or start a new orchestra. He didn't find a cure for childhood leukemia, either, or trek across the desert to rescue some orphans from an elephant stampede. Even being this year's drum major seems pretty un-phenomenal. I'm just trying to look at my son like an admissions officer, not as a mom who worships him. Really, he's just one more great kid among thousands.

The curtain will fall on September soon and the air is crisp as I limp to yoga today. I decide I'll take it easy, since my hips have been hurting; I have a lot of inexplicable pains. With all this yoga, I'd expect to feel a lot better than I have been lately.

As luck would have it (or possibly not) Jill announces that we're doing "hip openers." Don't ask me why or if this is a good thing, but when I mention that I've been having hip problems of late, Jill says this will help.

Weird that on the day the hip is bothering me most, Jill "coincidentally" devotes an entire session to that area. We recline on our backs and stretch our legs out to each side one at a time, using the belts to hold them in place for longer than usual. When I think I can't stand another second, Jill instructs, "Go to the breath," and as we do, she adds, "Now go deeper." Yes, that works, but I'm not sure if all this stretching is a good thing or not. I've been raised on traditional medicine, and I've made an appointment with my internist. But maybe I need to trust yoga when it comes to my health; it's certainly helped my head.

Just a few days later, my hip pain is almost completely gone and when I come to yoga I thank Jill for her help.

"I'm not surprised," Jill says, "but keep doing the poses at home so the pain won't come back."

She tells us today of going to hear the Dalai Lama. I'm so amazed by him, and the way Jill describes the experience— thousands of people, all coming together in complete silence to hear this man speak— makes me all the more in awe. In the paper today, I have read a letter by a local resident complaining of a neighbor who attends church in the morning and then goes to a Buddhist temple. You can't have it both ways, the writer says, chiding her neighbor for not "choosing" Christ. I can't imagine why one would have to choose between two men who carry the same message of peace and love. Obviously, this individual didn't absorb the message of either.

When I get home, the guidance counselor calls; she's done her homework and phoned three other school districts to see what their counselors advise. All say lie. She has also called admissions officers at three prestigious colleges. All say tell the truth.

I have to just laugh about this, since clearly adults don't have the answers. Yet kids are supposed to be perfect; and if they're not, we're expected to find a way to cover up their flaws. The way I see it, if colleges don't want kids with flaws, then they don't truly want real kids.

I thank her and hang up the phone, riffling through the college papers. I've promised Sam I'll call Carnegie Mellon University in Pittsburgh to make an appointment for him to attend a "sleepover weekend," so I dial the number and get an admissions officer on the line.

"Would your son like to stay in a Greek house?" she cheerfully inquires.

I envision Sam guzzling beer, smoking pot, and having sex with a co-ed in a toga: "A standard dorm will be just fine."

The last thing I want is for Sam to join a fraternity. I'm sure there are some perfectly innocent frats around, but when I was in college, the frat boys were the wildest, and the frat houses themselves reeked of drugs and alcohol. Of course, that was the Seventies, and all across America plenty of the *regular* dorms reeked of drugs and alcohol, too.

∞

September seems endless this year, though it's certainly a month I love. The applications still sit on my dining room table. The essays are still unwritten. All those statistics—how many years was the kid in band, how many AP courses, the SAT scores, the years, weeks, and months of volunteer work, on and on ad infinitum...are not yet answered.

I sit Sam down and remind him that this is not about *me*. "If you want to get into a good college maybe you should turn off the TV, stop I-M-ing friends, listening to music, running out for snacks, and answering your cell phone." Maybe, I add to myself, he should just stop living life.

In answer to my complaint, Sam spends the evening writing essays, whipping through four or five of them. As soon as he's finished, he asks, "Can I go out for a run with Gino? His chemo is over and he wants to celebrate! He may be coming back to school next month!"

It takes me a moment to realize he means a "run" for ice cream. Right now Gino, a star member of our track team, isn't up to taking a *real* run. Sam needs to study for his SAT II, and finish his regular homework. I think once again of how lucky we are to be able to go through this college application process, of how much or little it means to the future, and of how much I hope Gino, too, will be in college next year.

"Of course you can go."

CHAPTER SEVENTEEN: OCTOBER

Going with the Flow

My trip to the doctor about my recent hip problem is a waste of time, though I learn I have a bladder infection. My internist blows off my complaints as if I'm fantasizing; whatever is wrong—arthritis, bursitis, cancer—-must be my imagination. It almost seems as though in traditional medicine, if they can't figure out why you have pain somewhere, they simply deny that the pain exists. This isn't the first time a doctor has looked at me like I'm a lunatic because I have symptoms that can't be traced through blood or urine.

Sam and I sit down to begin the early decision Princeton application online tonight. Under the question "what language does your family speak at home?" Sam types in "pig Latin." Under "age and degrees of siblings," he types in that Ben, who is fourteen, has a PhD from Harvard. I'm glad to see he can have a sense of humor about this stuff. Of course, he hits delete after we're done laughing.

When he sees that I've edited his essays, though, he's rather pissed. "I don't like your ending," Sam argues. "Why did you change this one?"

"Everyone needs an editor or fact checker, and you're no exception," I explain. He takes on a lofty tone when he's writing, which is not like Sam at all. In a way it's too bad Ben can't write these essays—his prose has such natural rhythm!

After two hours of fiddling with the essays, it's nearly eleven. I drag myself to bed, and Sam runs out to meet a cute little redhead named Gretchen. I am totally wasted, but my son's night has just begun.

My doc has called with some lab results and apparently my cholesterol is high. There's so much heart disease in my family on my father's side, so this week I'm even more fixated on death than usual. After so many years of mistreating my body I wonder if I'll ever make up for the damage, no matter how much yoga I do. Thus, I'm in a grumpy mood when I set off for class. Yoga is just one more futile attempt to reverse the aging process.

Yet I also feel as if yoga may be a chance to restore my creaking structure, and when Jill suggests we dedicate our practice to something or someone, I decide to dedicate this practice to myself. I usually choose a friend in need or world peace or hurricane victims. But today, I honor my own health and future. Cheers!

I can keep up fairly well, but I feel somehow sad and hopeless, my mind wandering even as we go through the poses. I wonder if yoga *can* save a person, and if so, from what and how long does it take? Can it cure all those invisible fears as well as the aches and pains? Jill has gone to a lecture by B.K.S. Iyengar, the buff but elderly Indian "father" of modern yoga, who was a sickly child. He claims, basically, that yoga saved his life.

In a way, I feel as if the benefits of yoga are winding down for me. Perhaps I need to go deeper, not just in the poses, but in my thoughts about what yoga means. The whole first year was so new, so challenging. It seems that my impending winter doldrums have reached into my yoga practice, too.

∞

Sam and I are about to burst like balloons. I'm bursting because it takes so much energy not to pressure Sam, and he's bursting because he feels so pressured. I'd like to crash into his room, snap off his TV, sign him off of the IM, throw all his schoolbooks and CDs out the window, and just make him fill out the damn applications. But I can't do that. Because high school life marches on.

I notice that Sam's skin is acting up, and I make an appointment at the dermatologist. Of course, *my* skin is acting up, too. I'm fifty-two years old with the zits of a thirteen-year-old. If the Johns Hopkins researchers wanted to conduct an experiment about stress and pimples, mothers trying to help their kids get into college would be the perfect subject. I remember going through this process with Aaron; the day before deposits were due to be mailed, I actually had two checks written out to two different colleges because he couldn't decide. Eventually I proclaimed, "That's it, I'm mailing it to *this* one!" and when I saw his face fall, I mailed the deposit to the other. Just call me "Solomom."

Anneke stops by tonight carrying a bouquet of flowers and a hefty bottle of wine. As we settle in on the deck and raise our glasses she asks, "How is Sam coming along with his college applications?"

"Well, the portfolio isn't exactly coming together, and I can't figure out how kids who don't have architecture in high school are supposed to come up with one, anyway. And the interviews aren't really lining up, either. The essays, my God, you'd think these kids were trying to nab the Pulitzer Prize."

In the midst of our conversation, Sam wanders onto the deck and sits.

"So. What are your priorities?" Anneke asks. She's looking for a rundown of colleges, in order, of where Sam has applied and wants most to attend.

"To learn," Sam says without skipping a beat.

Anneke and I stare at one another, dumbfounded. Then we just shake our heads in shame.

Holding Patterns

Tonight, Sam is up late working on his architectural portfolio at the dining room table when I hear him yell, "Shit!"

I turn from my work in the kitchen to find blood spurting from his hand—there's a deep gash in his thumb. I rush him into the bathroom and wrap the injury with a bandage, but the blood just keeps spilling out. Surely he's going to bleed to death.

"I'll run him over to the ER," Mitch says, surveying the problem as he comes in the door from the Opera. How handy to have a spouse who arrives home at midnight dressed in a suit. No need for me to change out of my jammies.

At 2 a.m. they return with three stitches and a cumbersome bandage; just in time for Sam to conduct at the Montclair State College band festival tomorrow. Sam is undaunted, while I envision him collapsing from blood loss on the turf of Montclair before the eyes of several thousand people. "Why did his mother let him conduct?" the crowd will demand. "Because she's a pushy bitch who's forcing him to apply to an Ivy League college," the chorus will answer: "You know the type…she only cares about the kid getting ahead in life, not how happy he is."

Of course, that's not true, and I'm certainly not pushy; if anything I've always been a laissez-faire mom when it comes to making my children do things that they're hesitant to try. There's nothing I want more than happiness for my kids, just like every other parent I know. It's just that sometimes our motives get twisted up, and we become confused. We can't figure out if our kids will be happier if we push them harder or if we should just leave them the hell alone. I have a feeling that I'll never live it down if I let Sam slide through the fall of his senior year without giving the effort one hundred percent. But it's up to him.

In the morning, I watch a tape of Charlie Rose interviewing B.K.S. Iyengar that Jill has lent me. Rose keeps asking this great master why people do yoga, unabashedly admitting his total ignorance of the subject. Apparently, Mr. Rose is not a yogi kinda guy. For once, I feel pretty savvy.

After lunch, we all head out for the band festival. Sam conducts with style despite his bandaged thumb. Ben is in the marching band, too, playing the alto sax. I certainly seem to have a thing for musicians!

It's a dark, frosty morning in mid-November and we pack ourselves into the van at 3:30 a.m., bound for Pittsburgh, Pennsylvania, to explore the famed Carnegie (pronounced CarNEGie we learn) Mellon University. Sam is ready for the "sleeping bag weekend," which means, basically, that he'll sleep on the floor in one of the dorms, be granted an interview with an admissions officer, tour the campus, and get to talk to the students who attend the school. We're leaving Ben home with Aaron, and my mother-in-law has also come to help mind the fort.

I'm already prejudiced against CarNEGie Mellon, even though Holly Hunter and Ted Danson graduated from it, and even though it's the first totally wired campus in the nation. I'm prejudiced because at 3:30 in the morning, driving to Pittsburgh, Pennsylvania seems like an awfully tedious occupation. But, looking on the bright side, this must be the longest I've been in the presence of our busy boy Sam in months, and even though he's snoring I relish this time together.

Nearly seven hours later, we reach our destination, find a parking spot in a spacious garage, and hightail it to the information session, where the dean likens picking out a college to "choosing a bagel." Next, he goes on to a PowerPoint presentation featuring not only bagels, but pictures of tarts, croissants and Krispy Kreme donuts. Somehow his analogy is skewed. After all, if choosing a college were like selecting a bagel, then the visuals would just show a big basket of bagels. Maybe CMU would be the "everything" bagel, and a school like Princeton would be the garlic bagel (slightly esoteric, and only for really sophisticated kids) while Penn State would rank as the raisin bagel, just the sort of bagel that every kid loves to smother in cream cheese.

Instead, through my bleary eyed exhaustion, I'm wishing for some goddamn eggs. A college should provide some protein, in my opinion, whether it's in the form of an omelet or a class in physics.

At 5 p.m., we drop Sam at the student center where he's to meet his roommate for the night. Parents aren't allowed into the auditorium this time, so Mitch and I linger in the hallway, watching our son vanish into college life. Then we look at each other expectantly.

"Dinner?" Mitch asks.

"Sounds good to me."

We stroll to restaurant row, just a few blocks away from the campus, deciding on a reasonable Indian place. Delicious fare, but I'm so tired I can scarcely muster the energy to chew.

After dinner, we crash at a rundown motel on the outskirts of town. We shuffle inside with our bags and melt into a king-sized bed, which is so immense that I can't find my husband in it— and if I could, nothing would happen. I'm totally exhausted, stressed, and shocked by the realization that Sam will be leaving us, possibly to go as far away as Pittsburgh, PA, the ends of the earth.

As I snuggle into the pillow, Mitch reaches out to put his arms around me.

"I know where this is going," I snap, "and I'm too damn tired."

"*I* did all the driving. Why should *you* be so exhausted?" he turns and rolls to the far opposite side of the bed, so far away that I couldn't touch him, even if I wanted to. My husband is a very sensitive guy when it comes to sexual rejection.

I understand why he's miffed. We're finally alone in a motel room after twenty-two years of centering our marriage on our kids, and nothing is happening. But I just don't care. All I care about is whether Sam will insist upon going to CMU, and if he does, when and how I will ever see him again. I remember when he was a baby. We would sit in a rocking chair nursing, and Sam, with a mischievous grin, would invariably pull off his tiny fuzzy blue sock and flap it in my face. I sort of feel like that's what he's doing now.

I can't fathom how Mitch could think that this college trip would be a romantic get-away. He must be crazy to imagine that I'd feel joyful to be alone with him in a shabby Pittsburgh hotel while my son is doing God knows what on a nearby college campus (and possibly in a toga). I can't separate this evening from the knowledge that it's the beginning of our son's independence from us, while my husband views the trip as a fabulous excuse to be alone in a bedroom without teenaged boys down the hall.

If I haven't the energy for sex, I certainly don't have the

energy to argue, and Mitch can just be grumpy if he wants. I know from experience that grumpiness does eventually pass (usually in direct correlation to the next opportunity for romance). I reach my foot across the wide expanse and graze the tip of his ankle. But that's the best I can do; within moments, I'm out cold.

We awaken before seven and drive back to the university. Since nothing seems to be happening in the entire state of Pennsylvania, I'm amazed that the bumper-to-bumper traffic into Pittsburgh is worse than the commute from New Jersey to Manhattan. At the college, we nibble cold bagels (still no protein), drink tepid decaf, and await Sam. Eventually, he ambles down the hallway, his hair ruffled, eyes glazed. A slim blonde is at his side; hopefully, they haven't spent the night together.

On the way home, Sam chatters nonstop for a good fifteen minutes, then cuts us off, plugging his MP3 player into his ears. Apparently, he's enjoyed his night in the dorm, but the architecture students have warned him to steer clear of CarNEGie Mellon. It's too hard, they say. Run while you can. Go anywhere but here. Find an easy school, a school where you can have fun.

Not surprisingly, my son takes this as a challenge. "I like this place," he proclaims as we drive through the infinite void of Western Pennsylvania. "And hard work doesn't scare me."

∞

I enter yoga sheepishly, having missed class on Tuesday, and right away Jill cries out, "Where *were* you? Are you okay?"

"Mitch wanted to hang out together so I took class off," I explain, not going into the fact that I needed to use my female magic to make his male grumpiness pass.

"Oh! I understand," Jill nods with relief. It's strange that she's so worried.

Class is difficult today, and I find myself thinking, once again, of how much older I am than all these women. I doubt I'll be coming here when I'm sixty, keeping up with thirty-five or forty-year-olds. Which leads to the thought that maybe, some day, Jill will get married, have kids and give up teaching at least for a while. But before I go deeper down into this mind gully, I stop myself. The impermanence is all the more reason to treasure this time now, and make the most of what I *can* do. And besides, why *not* practice at sixty? Look at Iyengar, after all!

Jill begins with a chanting meditation, and I recall how shocked I was at my very first class more than a year ago, when Ali started with three repetitions of "Om" in unison. At the time, I thought this was an outlandish practice. Now, here I am chanting some Sanskrit words with my eyes closed and my index fingers and thumbs touching in Jnana mudra, as if this is a perfectly normal pastime, like weeding the garden.

During our practice, I try to accomplish everything that Jill instructs, even the hopeless "Dancer's pose," which looks so beautiful when she demonstrates, tipping forward with her right arm outstretched.

After class, I head out for the grocery store, where I run into the mom of one of Sam's peers. "Eddie and I are spending the day filling out college applications," she tells me. I feel rather envious. At least she'll be sitting down with her kid, talking, arguing, engaging in conversation. Since Sam's last application was mailed in early November, I've scarcely seen him at all. He's either at band, play practice, bowling, or Gretchen's house. When he *is* home, his door is closed, just as Aaron's was his senior year, just as mine was when I was seventeen, just as Ben's will one day be. The year before they leave for college, they're really already gone. Sometimes, I'm so melancholy thinking of this I just park myself outside Sam's room on the couch and read, hoping he'll snort a pleasantry (or even an insult) my way when he passes by to grab something from the refrigerator.

CHAPTER NINETEEN: DECEMBER

A Rather Large Puddle

I go to yoga today, even though I still have a cold. I've forgotten to bring a scrungie to tie back my hair, which I've been growing lately because Mitch likes it long, because I figure I won't want to have long hair when I'm really old, and because Robin from my wine club who cuts hair for a lot of money says I should. I suppose that's the *real* reason—not because my husband prefers it long. Now that a professional has told me to grow my tresses, I am.

Jill asks, "What do you *really* need? Do you need all the stuff that you own?" I think of all the Christmas items that will soon be filling my closets. Already, I've spent several hundred dollars on the kids, and I've just gotten started. The other day, I attempted to locate a sweater and couldn't find it because my drawers are so jam-packed with clothes—mostly clothes that I don't even wear but can't bear to part with. Yoga makes you think about some of the silly things we do in life, like collecting clothing and toys and other objects that we think will make us

154

happy, when the truth is, like the Little Prince said, everything that really means anything you can't touch.

I'm the first one to arrive this morning, and it's just Jill and me in the room for ten minutes before class. We like to talk about books—it turns out she's a prolific reader— and I find myself opening up to Jill more and more, telling her about Mitch and the kids, and she, in return, has begun to reveal a few things about her personal life, like the fact that she's been dating. With her looks and spirit, I'm sure that when she's ready to marry she'll just snap her fingers and the right guy will turn up. When Jill really wants something she simply "puts it out there," and the universe just seems to say to her, "Right back at ya."

Today Jill's subject is "coincidence," and it's clear that she doesn't really believe the popular adage that "shit just happens." I consider the fact that this yoga center opened a block away at a time when I really needed to take my life in a new direction. I'm not sure if this was coincidence or part of the master plan. I know Jill would say the latter, and so would many of my religious friends. I do agree that the more one pays attention to the way life's details sometimes fit together so perfectly, the more everything seems connected—just the way every asana is connected to the next, and every action has its complement, or counter action.

I meet with my writers' group tonight, and we laugh and share our kid problems and talk about our hopes for our manuscripts. When I consider whether it was coincidence that hooked me up with these women, I know it's something more, as if my muse looked down on me one day toiling in my little hovel of an office and mused (appropriately), "It's time to find this poor woman some wonderful writer friends." Not long after my muse made that observation, my friend Amy called and said she was starting a writers' group. She had two other women already lined up and wanted me to join.

We decided to keep it small, and we're not sorry. We're more like sisters now than anything else, and when we get together we have to catch up on family news. Our kids range in age from three to twenty-two, and we all have boys, so just keeping track of what's going on with our children can take up half of our meeting. "Remember, ladies…we're here to talk about our writing!" I have to remind. We talk about writing for ten more minutes, and then someone trails off on their kids. The little buggers just seem to get into everything—even when they're not here.

It's mid-December, only twelve days until Christmas, and my practice today is totally distracted. My problem is that I've been called back for a second mammogram. I can't help thinking morbid thoughts, and wondering why, at this time in my life when I'm living an increasingly healthy lifestyle, my body seems to be failing. I guess I've been hoping that yoga would be a quick fix. Hah!

On the other hand, this preoccupation with impending doom is making me realize how lucky I am. I love my kids, my husband, and my friends and family. I remember when my mother died, she just kept saying she was okay with death, but she didn't want to leave her family. I can't really say I'm okay with death, but I definitely understand the second part of her statement. Of course, my mother was religious in ways that I'm not, and so she had that solace.

In my restless state, I turn the wrong way in one of the poses, but when Jill corrects me I simply smile and make the adjustment. Usually, yoga takes me away from thoughts of gloom and fear, but today, it just isn't doing the trick. If I were to confront a real health crisis in my life, I'll bet yoga wouldn't be able to help much. Maybe it's good for back pain or a stuffy nose, but I can't see how these crazy moves could really make a difference in a crisis.

Yet, yoga does teach us to be in the moment, which Jill reminds us, is the only moment we have. When I'm philosophical about this, I realize that I have absolutely no power over the future, and that whatever is going to happen to me (or to anyone), has already been set in motion.

Apparently things *have* been set in motion for a long time. I spend the day at the mammography center in a heightened state of worry. Each time I sit down in the waiting room, I'm called back. "Just one more view," the technician promises, but then there's another, and another.

"You'll need a sonogram," she says next, leading me to a special room. And then it's, "A biopsy is required. We can do it here and now."

"This can't be happening," I'm thinking; it's probably one of those ludicrous mistakes I'll laugh and curse about later.

But the radiologist doesn't seem light-hearted, and when I mention that I'm nearing menopause and my breasts are probably just lumpy from old age she doesn't even smile.

"You'll need to have a portion of the right breast removed," she says grimly after the biopsy. She's detected a menacing lump that's not supposed to be there. Though she's sending the biopsy to a lab, the radiologist doesn't like what she's seen, and the urgency in her tone is ominous.

I try breathing; I try calming myself; I try being my best yoga self, but I am shaking and breathless and terrified. The nurse, whose name is Jill, whispers in my ear, "Why don't you call Dr. L…I'll give you her number. I'm not really supposed to offer an opinion, but she's the surgeon *I'd* call."

Why the hell is her name Jill? Talk about coincidences! She plants a book about breast cancer in my hands, and I nearly demand, "Why are you giving me *this?* I can't have breast cancer; that's absolutely preposterous!"

I dress in a daze and walk out into the clinic lobby. In all of my imagined fears, breast cancer has never been on my list; it doesn't run in my family, and I don't have any of the risk factors. I had my first child at the age of thirty, and I nursed all three, seemingly forever. It just figures that I'd end up with the one disease I never even worried about! I've always felt that my breasts—quite ample, but not oversized—were immune from any medical issues. They've always worked just fine.

When I return home, I tell Mitch about the experience.

"There must be a mistake," he says as he holds me in his arms. "I'm sure you're fine, so let's not jump to conclusions. Let's wait for the biopsy results."

We tread lightly around the house all night long. We won't tell the kids unless we know for sure that the biopsy is positive. (I find it darkly comical that a "positive" result can be a very bad thing.) I make an appointment with the physician "the new Jill" has suggested, first checking with my ob/gyn to be sure she concurs. "Dr. L is precisely the surgeon I'd recommend," my obstetrician says.

I turn on the news: eleven shopping days left until Christmas! I stumble to yoga, even while knowing I'll never make it through the class without crying. I'm the first one here, and Jill looks at me with alarm as I come toward her, as if she already knows what I'm going to say.

"I think I have breast cancer," I whisper to her as she puts her arms around me. "They found a lump, and now I'm just waiting for the results of the biopsy."

Jill hugs me close. "It will be all right. It *has* to be."

"I'm so afraid," I confide.

Several of the power yoginis enter the studio so we part and I place my mat in my usual spot. I settle in and close my eyes; I don't want to look at anyone—especially Jill. I'll burst into sobs if our gazes meet. Since she seems to know me so well without even trying, I'm quite certain that she's feeling my pain today. Jill is always instructing us to have compassion for others— and you can be sure that's because she feels it herself.

I try to concentrate in class, but I seem to be having an out-of-body experience. The other women are laughing and light in their movements, and I realize that all these faces are new to me, that none of these women have been here as long as I, even though most of them have practiced yoga elsewhere for years; I'm missing the women from my early classes. I'm even missing the power yoginis.

Jill is at my side as often as possible, and when I fold into Pigeon pose she touches my back, pressing into me as I weep softly. Her hands are so sure, and so quiet. Part of my crying has to do with my fear for my own future; the other part with my gratefulness for Jill in my life. Coincidence or fate, I do believe I am *meant* to know Jill, and to have yoga to help me.

I'm to meet with the recommended surgeon today. Mitch has an important performance, and he expects good news anyway, so we decide that he won't take off. I've phoned Beth, and she's determined to come with me, even though I tell her I can go it alone.

"No way," she says, "I'll pick you up at 3:30 sharp."

Like Anneke, she's a nurse as well as my friend, after all, so she picks me up and we drive to the doctor's office. I think of the day, forty-some years ago, when Beth and I, then seven years old, purposely jumped into a deep, wide puddle on our way home from school. Black branches swayed in the water, reflected from the towering oak trees above; clouds drifted across its center and crows called from its icy-cold depths. We stood at the edge as if we were about to dive into a lake, and then gradually, clutching at each others' wrists, we entered, shyly at first, then splashing and stomping, falling onto our knees and then rising, wet to the bone. When we got to my house, my mom cried, "What on earth happened?"

"We *fell* in a big puddle!" I fibbed, and we ran upstairs to change our clothes, giggling our heads off.

But today we're not laughing, and once inside the office, I tell Beth, "Wait for me here." I feel that I need to be one-on-one with this doctor, so Beth reluctantly takes a seat and I'm ushered to the examining room.

Dr. L is a middle-aged woman, probably a tad older than I. She's just a tiny bit plump, with a soft, motherly gaze and an easy smile. Her hands on my breasts are gentle, and as they move over each inch and portion, I close my eyes and soak in the beauty and silence of her touch. I've never had a breast exam like this one— so cautious, so quiet— and I can tell this is a woman who will take the time I will need. I feel a lightness inside as she touches me, and I know that I've come to the right place. I notice that she's wearing a pretty shade of pink nail polish, but the color is chipped. She's a woman who cares about her hands, but uses them well and often.

After the exam, Dr. L sits next to me on the examining table, folds her arms around me, and tells me I have cancer. She has already reviewed my lab report from the mammography center, and knows for sure. We discuss some of the details, but not all. I won't know more until I have an MRI.

I feel as if I'm living fiction; it's frightening to know this is fact.

Dr. L rests her hand on my arm. "If all goes well," she says, "and if the MRI confirms my suspicion that the cancer hasn't spread, I can remove the lump and you will then be treated with chemotherapy and radiation. The chances of survival here are high."

Her voice is very soft and her tone sounds hopeful, but I don't want to hear the word "survival" at all. There can be no *question* of it, even if the chances are good.

"How long has the lump been there, do you think?" I ask, expecting her to say it's a recent development. After all, I go for an annual check up.

"I'd guess about five years. It often takes that long before a tumor is large enough to be detected on the mammogram," Dr. L explains.

"I had no idea."

I share the results with Beth when I come out of the office, and she calms my tears as we drive home. "Don't go down that road!" she orders when I start predicting the future, but we both know this is the road I've followed all my life—the path of negativity and fear, the road that I've been trying to get off ever since I first came to yoga. I think about the day I didn't want to pick up Beth's laundry. Now, she's here with me, offering comfort, urging me to stay strong and positive.

From the car, I call Mitch on my cell; it's intermission, and for once, he's left his phone on. He's shocked by my news. "We'll get through this," he says with authority.

Beth drops me home, and I thank her for coming with me; then I step inside, pausing in the foyer for a moment to brace myself before telling the boys. "Guys! I need to talk to you all a moment!" I call as I head for their bedrooms, and within seconds they all convene in the hallway, for once, obeying without hesitation. Something in my tone must warn this won't be a conversation about picking their dirty clothes up off the floor.

"I've gone for my yearly mammogram," I explain, "and a cancerous lump has been found. I'll need surgery to have it removed." My voice breaks as I deliver this information, but I try to maintain control. I don't want them to know how scared I am; I don't want to share the fear that's coursing through my body.

Sam blinks back tears, but Aaron puts his arm around me and gives me a hug.

"You'll be fine!" he assures me.

Ben, I don't think, will let me know how he feels, although I can tell he's frightened. He's at an age when feelings can't always be shown, though they're as strong as the winds of a hurricane.

When I come downstairs the phone is ringing. Jill is on the line; this is the first time she's ever called me, and I feel peace as soon as I hear her voice.

"I want you to be positive," she urges. "I want you to use your yoga, and I *promise*—I will help you handle this. You are going to be all right."

∞

Sam is deferred at Princeton today, the day after I'm informed I have breast cancer. That sort of puts everything in perspective. An Ivy League college is marvelous, but it sure ain't the end all.

I'm happy he hasn't been outright rejected, so at least there's hope. And hope is a good thing.

So we're in waiting mode now, and we won't know about Sam till spring. And I'm in waiting mode, too. Waiting and hoping.

I make all the necessary phone calls to my various friends and relations, guilty and depressed to have to say these words; that I have to ruin my sister's afternoon, and send my brother into gloom, and make all my friends cry and worry. But there's just no other way since they'll find out eventually. In my family we like to put all our cards out on the table—after all, we've been raised to *expect* this kind of news.

Anneke, being the nurse that she is, wants to discuss my treatment.

"I can't go there right now," I say. "I'll have to take this one day, one hour at a time."

"I understand completely. But I just want you to know there may be a little discomfort after the surgery…and chemo often causes hair loss."

"I don't give a shit about my hair," I shoot back. "I just want to live."

"That's my girl," Anneke says.

On the weekend, Mitch and I drive into the City for lunch. As we pull into a parking spot, I remember that Eloise is in this neighborhood with her son today. Each Saturday she or her husband drives to Manhattan from upstate New York to bring Jeb to Mannes College The New School For Music for bassoon and composition lessons. I rifle through my bag, searching for her cell number, cursing myself for not programming it into my phone. Oddly, I find a slip of paper with a number in the bottom of my purse— it looks like a possibility.

Turns out it's her son's number, left over from a day on the Cape when Eloise was borrowing his cell. He's left the phone in her car, but just as I call, she's retrieving a book from the back seat, and hears it ringing. Normally, she tells me, this phone is never left on. And anyway, she can't imagine why I still have her son's number in my handbag.

We meet on the corner of Amsterdam Avenue and 87th Street and hug and hug and hug. It's raining and we're crying; we're Audrey Hepburn and George Peppard at the end of Breakfast at Tiffany's, only we don't kiss on the lips and there's no mewling cat between us.

∞

I've had a few sleepless nights. I remember what Jill said at one of our very first classes: "Imagine the best outcome, then the worst, then go to the middle." I'm trying to stay in the middle, to stay centered and strong.

I go to yoga today, since I don't know when I'll be able to practice again, and I want to see Jill and Natalie and update them. They both throw their arms around me when I come in, and Natalie suggests some books about visualization. In the past I would have scoffed at this, but now I welcome the idea. I'll try anything and everything I can.

I'm expecting yoga to be just too hard today, but instead I breeze through the poses, basking in how I can move and control my body. How strange to think that a part all along has been doing its own thing, and not in a good way. Maybe this is what my body has been trying to tell me for months—too bad I wasn't listening.

When I get home, the phone rings and a cheery nurse informs me that my MRI will be tomorrow, as if I've just won the Pick Five in the lottery. I've gotten some Xanax from Dr. L, and Mitch is taking off work; I don't know which is worse— my fear of what the MRI results will show or my fear of lying motionless in an enclosed space for more than half an hour.

I straighten some papers and pack away my Christmas cards— there's no way I can deal with them now. But at the last moment, I pluck one out to send to Winston, a "boy" who now lives in New England, with whom I've been friends since fourth grade. If Winston didn't hear from me, he'd surely think I was dead since this is an annual ritual we've been following for decades. I don't want to put that particular notion out into the universe, so I send a card to my dear childhood friend; the rest can wait.

Surprise, surprise, the MRI went swimmingly, not that lying on my stomach with my boobs dangling while peering into what looked like a fish bowl was a joyride. But all things considered, it wasn't so bad. Sure beats a sharp stick in the eye, as one of my newspaper editors used to say.

But now I'm in waiting mode, and my wandering mind takes paths that I'd rather not explore. After dinner, I hop in my car and drive to a yoga classmate's—she's called to offer a free session in some kind of New Agey healing energy therapy. In her office, I toss balls back and forth, stare at red patches of color, twirl a magic wand in my fingers, and make arc-like motions with my arms while repeating the names of my closest relatives. Each time I come to Virginia, my mother, something strange seems to happen: I burst into tears; I drop the ball; I sigh with regret. Could this all possibly be about my mother? I've read that women who experience trauma or stress are more likely to get cancer.

My classmate sits scribbling notes in a corner, glancing up now and then to suggest another move for me to try. She must think I'm a real "case," but in this line of "energy work" I'm sure she sees plenty of women with "issues." Why else would they be tossing balls and twirling magic wands?

When I step out of the office, I'm somehow lighter, but also depressed. I feel as if I've finally let my mother go. But what am I left with? Breast cancer. What a lovely trade.

∞

I practice my Downward Dogs and Cobras and Tree in my bedroom today and imagine that my immune system sparks up with each motion. I bake a pumpkin pie from scratch and then an apple pie.

I call Dr. L but she has no results. More waiting, more wandering in my thoughts to the future and then trying to ground myself again. It's as if I'm pacing inside my own head, up and down the corridors of my mind, trying to keep the doorways to despair from opening. I don't want to think of what will happen if the MRI shows the cancer has spread. I don't want to think of all the things that might be on the road ahead if there is lymph node involvement or cancer detected in my other breast.

Mitch goes out for a jog, but I'm here waiting by the phone. I feed the birds in my yard and breathe. The sky seems incredibly vast—wider and more mysterious than ever.

Two days until Christmas. Dr. L calls with the MRI results; no other problems are apparent, so we will go ahead with the lumpectomy as discussed. This is fantastic news and for a day I'm almost jubilant. Mitch and I hug and grin at one another, our hearts full of hope. In spite of the cold, we walk, we eat out, and I try to look at everything afresh.

By Christmas Eve, I'm miserable as hell. I can't believe *this* is Christmas. My brother, his wife, and my nephew arrive as well as Mitch's sisters and mom. I smile and serve food, but I can't wait until the holiday is over. I'm not in the moment, not at all, and when I look into my relatives' faces, all I see is worry.

Christmas Day is slightly better, after a sleepless night. I'm busy with the meal preparations; as I wash the cranberries, I gaze deeply at their color and feel the hard nodules of their flesh between my fingers. I am *in* the cranberries; I'm a little red cranberry myself. I'm trying my best to keep my thoughts on what I am doing in the now. This is not an easy task; I realize I've never really tried it before— and it never seemed to matter so much.

I never considered my mind to be such an enemy; I've

been brought up to believe in intelligence and thoughts. Now I'm trying to fling my thoughts away because they're repetitive, negative, and have so much more to do with the past or future than the present. It's actually amazing I've lived *this* long with thoughts like these!

After the relatives leave, I focus on cleaning up the kitchen, putting the presents away, and erasing the happy trail of Christmas faster than I ever have before. Still, I'm looking forward to returning to yoga tomorrow.

In the morning, I email two of my favorite cousins; we constantly played together as children—we loved to be rock stars, using the removable wooden spindle from my parents' four-poster bed as our microphone. I didn't want to tell them before Christmas; I thought it might be too upsetting, and it's not as though we see each other very often so there's no rush. My female cousin, who has the same sweet nature and walnut-brown eyes as my mom, is shocked and worried, but her brother writes that I have stout genes, and he'll send me a male stripper. I adore them both.

At yoga, Jill talks about angels today—about friends who visit our lives for a reason— and I know she is one.

I head home after class, but then, on a whim decide to keep walking, trying to notice every detail along my path. I've been reading and re-reading *The Power of Now* by Eckhart Tolle, and I admit that when I am in the "now," I feel lighter. When I listen to the birds lined up like abacus beads on the telephone wires, and notice the jet stream of an airplane or the blue of the sky overhead, my heart lifts. I don't want to be worrying about breast cancer, or any cancer. I want to be living my life.

Just two more days until the New Year. Before class today, Jill whispers, "I've been focusing on you, trying to come up with ways I can help!"

Doesn't she know how much she's helped already? She's the one who got me thinking about living in the present moment. Until yoga, I never even realized I wasn't in it.

Last night, Mitch encouraged me to imagine white blood cells traveling to the cancer site, and to meditate on the location of healing. Instead of white cells, I thought of white roses, then white daisies, then white horses and white unicorns. Every time my thoughts turn to cancer, I rest on the couch, place my hands on my breast, and send the roses, daisies, horses and unicorns. I know this is wacky stuff, but at least it's not hurting. I throw in some white bunnies and adorable angora kittens for good measure.

In yoga today, I tone everything down. I can't hold my Handstand prep for a full minute as the others can, and I don't mind. I am different from them; now, more than ever. But I do manage to stay in a Downward Dog for a full minute, and I can't help but think that yoga will keep me strong. I can't imagine not being able to practice during my recovery. But hey, just as long as there *is* a recovery, I'll deal.

The holiday weekend is approaching, but that doesn't stop hospitals from doing their work. Eloise drives down from upstate New York and accompanies me to my pre-op testing. She asks me what she can do.

"I want to help you," Eloise says, as we wait outside the testing rooms. "I want to be a good friend. Tell me what I can do; tell me what you need from me now."

"Just be yourself," I say, and she puts her arms around me and starts to cry.

I'm glad she's with me because the male nurse who gives me

my EKG appears to be wearing a funky black toupee, and he seems to speak mostly Russian. The thought of being alone in the room with him with my boobs unveiled sort of freaks me out, but with Eloise nearby reading her bunny book— *Watership Down*— it seems okay. I'm nervous about the results of the blood tests and my chest x-ray. But having Eloise here helps me to be in the moment, because I love being with her so much. Waiting next to someone you love is much easier than waiting alone; just being together is a gift—there's no such thing as "just passing the time" any more.

Anneke stops in tonight already in tears; as soon as I open the front door, she throws her arms around me.

We settle in at my dining room table to talk. "Do you have someone you could discuss this with?" I ask. "Someone *other* than me? Maybe your pastor?"

It seems ironic that I'm trying to be supportive of her, when I'm the one with breast cancer, but that's just the way it is. Anneke, for all her outward joking and theatricality, is a soft and fragile woman on the inside. She could really benefit from a big fat dose of positive yoga philosophy; she seems to see everything from the dark side, even though (or possibly because?) she's a fervent Christian.

"I'm sorry," Anneke apologizes, dabbing her tears. "I just can't help it."

We chat for a few moments about the kids and politics and then she takes her leave. I think she's just come to "check up on me," though it seems that maybe *she's* the one who needs looking in on. But even though I love Anneke like a sister, I don't really want to see how my illness is upsetting her; I have to take care of myself, and that means staying positive. Tears are fine, but if everyone around me starts weeping when they see me, I won't be able to take the steps I need. Mitch calls himself my "mood stabilizer," and I believe he's right; the man just seems to inspire level-headedness. But whenever I see Anneke I get a different feeling—as if she doesn't really believe I'm going to make it.

It's New Years Eve, strange but true, and the kids are all out at parties. Mitch is upstairs practicing, so I'm alone once Anneke leaves. I roll out my mat, and as soon as I begin to move, I feel stronger. I have to remember that when I'm feeling weak, and when my mind goes down those unhappy pathways, I can guide myself into the present and renew myself with yoga.

Well, happy New Year. I *hope* it's a happy year. I can face whatever is ahead of me, as long as I'm alive.

CHAPTER TWENTY: JANUARY

Wandering as I Wonder

Crazy things are happening. Ruthann sends me a pink beaded bracelet she bought a month ago from a woman who was raising money for breast cancer. I open a book I notice on a shelf and find a breast cancer bookmark. I read a story for a proofreading job and it's about breast cancer. Maybe there have been a million little signs even before these that I've been missing.

What could have caused it? White wine, hair dryers, deodorant, peanuts, my coffee bean grinder which sends a nasty electric current up your arm when you press it with your finger, underwire bras, decaffeinated coffee, chicken or beef pumped with hormones, our drinking water... I wonder if it could be something as stupid as sleeping on my stomach? Like SIDS. Women who snore on their breasts are bound to get it? SIBS... Sudden Instant Breast Syndrome. *Gotcha!*

I concentrate on all the strong women who have survived breast cancer: Elizabeth Edwards, Melissa Etheridge, and a couple of women from town. I don't want to think of the ones who have lost the "battle." I don't even want to acknowledge that it *is* a battle.

Is it a "bump in the road," as my cousin says? I hope he's right. But what a bump…the kind that sends you soaring up to smash your head on the car ceiling when you speed over it. A bump is a lump, is a nasty hump in the road with a toad, as Dr. Seuss might say.

I've told most of my friends and that part is getting easier. I was so consumed with dread I could hardly get my words out when I made those first phone calls, but today I find myself comforting a former neighbor and reassuring a friend from my brunch club. It will be all right, *I'm* telling *them* now. It had better be.

We've been warned by the guidance counselors to fill out the FAFSA (the form that parents have to complete if they want financial aid) early, so we do. It takes two hours, even with a worksheet, because every time I make a mistake the file automatically returns me to the beginning. When it's complete, I hastily check my email, and there's an urgent notice about erectile dysfunction. Mitch, peering over my shoulder, asks with alarm, "What the hell is that doing on the FAFSA?" He's such a computer-savvy guy.

There's nothing more to do except wait for the colleges to respond. Sam has already gotten into all his "safety" schools, so we know he's going *somewhere*. We'll have to wait for the biggies, and it's a damn good thing because I don't think I can focus on Sam's bright future right now. I just hope and pray that I'll be here in four years when he graduates, and that I'll be able to see Ben through his own college application process. It's amazing how the activities that have annoyed me this fall now seem like incredible privileges. Jill is so right; the little challenges we meet every day are part of what makes life interesting. I'm not so sure about the big challenges, though, especially the one called cancer. I could live quite happily and gratefully without having to face up to *that* in my life.

∞

My second to last yoga class before the surgery. "I don't know when I'll be back," I moan to Jill as I place my mat on the floor.

"Just come and sit; you don't have to do the asanas. Just come," she suggests.

That seems silly to me, but maybe I'll miss her words so much, I'll want to. She is the wisest thirty-something-year-old I've ever known.

In class, I push myself, going for the stretches and lunges, holding my Planks, pushing into my Downward Dog. I don't know if I should be taking it easy, acting like a person who is sick. I don't *feel* sick; I feel stronger than I ever have in my life.

During Savasana, Jill stops by my mat and places her hands on my feet, runs them across my thighs. Then I sense heat just above my forehead, and I know that she's doing some kind of healing magic. Everyone's eyes are closed, of course, and no one knows that this healing voodoo is directed just at me. I've been chosen for a great honor, for an award, as if I'm the child who's been selected class president.

Later, I set out for a hair cut, just a trim to get me through the next few weeks (possibly, before all my hair falls out from chemo). I tell my hairdresser, Irene, about my problem, and she starts crying. It's amazing how much love I'm collecting from my world.

I thought I was awake before, but this is one hell of a caffeine jolt. I wasn't even half awake, I'm finding. I wonder if the universe remembers that I'm allergic to caffeine—one sip of the stuff and I break out in awful hives. "Hey out there—you can wake me up with a mellow cup of decaf—I don't really need the cosmic espresso special!"

∞

My last yoga class…for a while. I give Jill a journal as a present and a dream journal to Natalie, because she is a woman of many dreams. They open their gifts and hug me, but we're all too emotional for words. Natalie hands me a piece of paper— the name and number of a friendly yogic "competitor" nearby who specializes in yoga and health issues. "Call her," Natalie urges, tucking the paper into my hand.

Somehow I make it through the class, though today I feel weak and vulnerable. I let myself take Child's pose when the others are still in their Handstands, but I do manage a Headstand—relish it, even—not knowing when I'll be able to do one again. It's funny to think that doing a Headstand or Handstand could have meant so much to me. Now I'm much more concerned with how yoga can help me stay healthy and strong. "Safe" and "strong" are the words that keep coming into my thoughts today. Safe and strong.

I try not to dwell on the possibility that this may be my last class for the foreseeable future, even while Jill's sweet hands pass over me during Savasana, even while I feel them hovering above me again, sending me healing vibrations. But after class, on the way out, I burst into tears, hugging both Natalie and Jill, thanking them for all they've given me. Another student joins us, and it turns out she too is experiencing a breast cancer scare, although she hasn't been diagnosed. She is scheduled for an MRI next week, and we put our arms around one another. She's a stunning, svelte brunette who I've never talked to one-on-one. Today we are crying in each other's arms.

Breast cancer and yoga. Unlikely partners. You wouldn't think that women who do yoga would get any kind of cancer, ever. But here we are, and now we have to figure out what to do.

Here *I* am, anyway.

As soon as I get home I call the yoga teacher Natalie has recommended, a woman named Jeanine, who has worked with breast cancer survivors. She's not in, so I leave a message. How is it possible that less than a mile from my home is a yoga teacher who may know exactly what I need? "In yoga," as Jill says, "there are no coincidences."

I make dinner for Mitch and the boys, who seem to be acting as if it's just "business as usual." But it feels as if there's an inaudible hum accompanying all my movements, and I sense that they're watching closely to see how I'm dealing with this. It's well-known by parents that when *we* freak out, our children get really worried—that's why it's a good idea to act nonchalant even when your kid falls off his bike and rises up bathed in blood with bones poking out in the wrong directions: "Oh, honey, I think we might just make a little trip to the ER. Nothing serious of course!"

After we eat, I head out with my writers' group for cappuccino to celebrate my upcoming birthday. We settle in around a small table at a local coffee shop, leaning toward each other to chat.

"How are you feeling emotionally?" inquires Jessica, an inveterate reporter who isn't afraid to ask any question.

"You know, the odds are all in your favor!" notes Kayla, whose husband is a physician.

"You're going to be just fine!" Amy says. This touches me more than anything, since she usually looks on the bleak side (strangely enough, yet another Presbyterian). She's making a Herculean effort to be positive, just for me, and the way they're all in enthusiastic agreement suggests that they've had a serious powwow on the way to pick me up, which makes me love them all the more. They think I am strong!

We order cake (it's my birthday, after all!), and Kayla places a basket on the table. Inside are warm, comforting gifts: fuzzy pink socks, a delicate nightgown, hand creams, teas, a fleecy, pink shawl and slippers. It's our habit to celebrate birthdays in this way; everyone pitches in and adds a gift. It helps that Kayla and Amy share the same birthday, though they are years apart in age. But three times a year we make a point of spoiling one another. Tonight it seems that there's extra spoiling going on.

We kiss and hug when they drop me at my house; we can't stop hugging.

I climb into bed in my new nightgown, with my shawl around my shoulders and my pink socks on, and I feel absolutely embraced by the warmth of their love.

∞

This morning, I reach Jeanine, the teacher Natalie suggested, and we chat on the phone for fifteen minutes; she has a class I can come to as soon as I'm ready.

Jeanine asks me to tell her about myself, so I describe my family, my friends, my writing. "When you go into surgery, I want you to think of all your friends holding hands and encircling you with love. Imagine that they're standing around the table, surrounding you with their best wishes and prayers for your health."

I adore that image—all my Republican and Democrat friends—forced by love of me—to make nice and hold hands!

I receive a beautiful card in the mail from Jill today—a drawing of a woman standing in Tadasana, finding her "mountain." I place it in a picture frame and hang it on my wall.

Then I decide to henna my hair, since one day not too long from now, I may not have any hair to henna. I sprinkle some henna into a bowl, add an egg, hot water and stir. It's a messy job, but I'd rather pour eggs than chemicals on my head, especially now. Walking around my house with my hennaed hair under a plastic bag, I imagine myself bald. The vision isn't pretty, and I'll be happy to see my auburn tresses in an hour.

Just as I'm shampooing the last bits of muck from my hair, Anneke stops in. "How about a cup of tea?" I offer.

"Sure!" she agrees. I boil the water while Anneke sits in her usual spot at my dining room table. I can't remember a time when Anneke and I didn't drink wine together, but none for me tonight; I want to be as toxin-free for my surgery as possible. This is a true sign of friendship, when someone who loves her Pinot Grigio will settle for a cup of decaf Earl Grey just to be with you. We raise our cups and toast to good health.

After Anneke leaves, I scurry into my office to check out some chat boards about surgery. The women on the web trade tips on what kind of bra to wear afterwards (soft) and give advice about what to bring to the hospital (warm socks, a button up blouse). I'd rather read about this than learn of my odds and chances. It's a comfort to click on the entries of women who have been there, done that, and lived to tell the tale.

I check on the boys — they're all busy with their homework, except Aaron, who now goes to sleep by ten for his early commute to the City—and then I settle into bed. I've been looking forward to this moment all day—not so that I can sleep, but so I can finally meditate and visualize. I have an important appointment with my "inner healer," a skinny older man with a long white beard who wears a dark purple robe with white velvet trim. He lives in a beautiful garden where he raises only white flowers—dogwood, lilacs, lilies, roses, and daisies. Sometimes he makes it snow in great, pelting flakes. With a wave of his hand, he dispatches the white doves, white unicorns and white horses, and every now and then he shoots my body with a wand of white light. I love lying on my couch or in bed imagining this man. I don't know why I haven't chosen a woman, but for some reason my inner healer is male; he reminds me of Gandalf in *Lord of the Rings*. I imagine myself, dressed in a gauzy white gown, with sparkling white flip-flops on my feet, and white baby's breath threading through my hair. I take my time watching myself walk down the winding staircase to the private garden, lit by miniature white lights. I'm even wearing white polish on my toe- and fingernails. When I arrive at the garden, I settle on a bench while he calls out his healing forces, and I lift up a white kitten or bunny to hold on my lap while my personal healer does his work.

I'd rather be lost in the white light and healing magic of my own imagination than predictions in a medical book.

My surgery is tomorrow. Ruthann has arrived on the sister express from North Carolina, and she's been making me laugh, and bringing me tea, and just being the familiar comfort of family. Being around Ruthann is like having a vase of fresh flowers permanently at my side. "I have only positive expectations for how this will go," she assures me often.

Natalie calls from the center and offers to lead us in a healing meditation. "Sure!" I say, "Come on over!"

A few minutes later, Natalie is at my door. She's brought her own CD player and she pops in a calming, New Age CD as we nestle under blankets on my living room floor. We close our eyes as Natalie leads us to a quiet, healing place, where we imagine we are soothed and protected; her gentle voice guides us through meadows and along a brook, with sunlight following our footsteps.

When we're done I thank Natalie for her kindness. At the door she turns to me: "Oh! I almost forgot!" She takes my hands in hers and shows me how to press my thumbs to my fingers, repeating "Sa, Ta, Na, Ma," at each pause. "This," Natalie explains, "will help you when you're afraid."

I glance at Ruthann, who's nodding in agreement, and I wonder if these wacky women in my life are witches or heavenly saints.

My friends who pray are praying for me, and my friends who send positive thoughts are sending their thoughts, and the air seems to be tingling and vibrating with all the love that is in my life. I have a moment of despair tonight, clinging to Mitch and crying, but when it's over I feel that I'll be safe and strong in the hands of my surgeon, with the thoughts and prayers of my friends vibrating my universe, which it turns out, is much bigger and wider than I ever knew.

This is the scariest day of my life. I pull on some sloppy, comfortable sweats, a button-down sweater and my pink socks, watch enviously while Ruthann and Mitch eat a yummy-smelling oatmeal concoction for breakfast, and kiss my kids good-bye. I wonder if I'll be alive at the end of the day; I can't help thinking of all the weird stories I've heard over the years of people going in for a little facelift, and never waking up. I try to envision my surgeon's healing hands. She doesn't *seem* like a woman who will screw up.

It's just a little tumor, after all. Hopefully, like its owner, it hasn't done a lot of traveling.

Mitch drives us to the hospital, my sister and I chatting nervously all the way there. My husband always wonders how Ruthann and I can talk so much—when we're together we never shut up. On the way, I remind my husband, "Please keep your cell phone on today. I don't have mine with me." I know my brother will be trying to get in touch.

Inside the hospital, I check in at the desk and a nurse hands me a shift and leads me to a tiny changing area. Next, a technician pops in to accompany me to an examining room; this, perhaps, is the worst part of the day's ordeal—a dye that is injected through a wire inserted in my breast. The blue dye will guide my surgeon to the sentinel lymph node (which sounds like some sort of lookout post, and indeed it is). The node will then be removed and sent to the pathology lab; if there's cancer in the sentinel node then there's a good chance it's in other nodes as well, but if the head honcho node is clear, then the others will be clear, too.

As the dye enters, my chest explodes with excruciating pain. It will be fun to be sliced by the surgeon instead of slowly tortured by this radiologist! I press thumbs to my index fingers, then to my middle, ring, and pinkies, silently repeating the chant Natalie taught me: "Sa, Ta, Na, Ma." I don't even know what this means; I only know that it calms me. I breathe, and follow my breath with my mind, reassuring myself that I have the skills and the strength to deal with this. I can't imagine how I would have gotten through this day without yoga, yet I haven't taken a single pose.

By one o'clock my blood sugar is dropping but pre-surgery snacks aren't allowed; I'm delivered back to the pre-op room where Ruthann and Mitch are waiting.

"Well, that was pretty terrible," I sigh as I come in. "I feel like I've just been stabbed by a vicious pirate! I wonder how the rest of the day will go!"

Ruthann and Mitch exchange glances and my sister nods at my husband. "Go ahead, tell her," she urges.

"Tell me what? I already know I have cancer," I answer wearily.

"Uh...there was a phone call while you were in that other room just now."

"What *kind* of a phone call?" I ask suspiciously.

"Now, don't be alarmed. It's nothing serious," Mitch says, "but the school nurse called. Sam's been hit in the head with a hockey stick!"

"*What?*"

"Yeah, some kid was screwing around in gym, and Sam got nailed. But he's going to be okay—I called Beth and she's driving him to the ER for stitches."

"*This* ER?"

"Yep."

Weirdly enough, we all start laughing! In our anxious state, it strikes us as funnier than hell that a mother can't get center stage in her own family even when she's undergoing breast cancer surgery.

At 2 p.m., I kiss my husband and sister, and a nurse leads me to the operating room. Outside the door, I burst into tears. It's not so much the fear itself as the sight of that table; the last time I was on something like that was for a happy occasion, for giving birth. The road from my last delivery— Ben, fourteen years ago—flashes before me. How could I have gotten here? How can a mother have to experience this? And yet, so many do. So many women, so many mothers have gone down this road before me.

As I climb onto the table, the nurses try to make me laugh. A lovely anesthesiologist who stopped by earlier to introduce herself, asks me what I like to eat and where I like to vacation; I suppose she's trying to distract me while she waits for me to drift away. Dr. L comes in, smiling as she bends near, and I realize that she must think I'm a horrible fool, lying here crying when she hasn't even begun to operate!

"I'm sorry to be such a baby," I sob. There it is again: the word "baby." It makes me sob even more.

I think of Ruthann, who is now wearing my pink wooly socks. I pulled them off my feet and made her put them on just before they brought me to the operating room (the nurse offered me some cozy hospital socks to replace them). The women in my writers' group are all wearing pink socks in my honor, and my book group has declared this fuzzy sock day for me. I try to focus on all my friends in their fuzzy socks, on my Republican friends, and my Democrat friends, who now I think of simply as the people who love me, the people I love. I imagine that they're all holding hands, encircling me as I drift away. I remember the circle of girlfriends who joined hands and sang a hymn around Eloise's mom's casket. But my friends are willing me to live, not sending me off to the afterlife.

Three hours later, I awaken. Dr. L is at my side, smiling brightly. "Things have gone well! The preliminary findings show no spread to the lymph nodes."

"Thank you Dr. L and thank you Jesus!" I sigh, adding the disclaimer that I'm really not religious. I don't even know why that Jesus thing popped out, but just in case, it can't hurt to say "thank you."

I do believe in prayer, though, and in all those healing thoughts, and the "Oms" that have been sent my way. I have to believe that some power keeps watch, because, as Billy says, "there has to be."

"Your urine may be a little blue from the dye for a while but not to worry," Dr. L says as she pats my arm.

I'm surprised that I'm alert enough to quip, "That's okay. I'm a liberal."

I spend some time in the recovery room; I'm groggy, but the pain isn't bad, and should it kick up I have a prescription for later use. Ruthann and Mitch peek in, and a kindly nurse watches over me. In just a few hours we're on our way home.

Of course, I'm thrilled to see my little house as we drive up the block—as if I've been on a trek in the wilderness instead of away at the hospital for one day. Inside, Aaron, Sam and Ben hug and kiss me as I come in the door. Ben's neck is crooked, and he's bent like a little old man with severe osteoporosis. He, too, has had an incident in gym class— hit while playing dodge ball. Sam's eye is red and bulging; there's a band-aid over his seven stitches and he resembles Mel Brooks' young Frankenstein. My boys are the reflections of my day; only Aaron seems to have escaped (I guess the lesson here is get a pass out of phys ed class when your mom's having surgery).

The house is brimming with flowers. On the dining room table is a gorgeous bouquet of white roses.

"Who sent these?" I ask the kids, searching for a card.

"We don't know, Mom," Sam replies. "They were stuck in the doorway when I came in, so I just put them in some water."

"Wow, they're beautiful," Ruthann says, touching the petals, and breathing in the scent.

I collapse in a chair and sigh with relief; I'm just so glad to be home.

Today is my birthday. How incredibly bizarre! A year ago I was at yoga class and Ali and the others were serenading me. Today, I'm *really* celebrating being alive.

I solve the mystery of the white roses. On the floor, I find a card from Jill: "Wishing you white light all day." Funny, because white light is exactly what I've been envisioning, coursing through my body. The roses are a little more open today, and they remind me of what Jill always says: "Open your heart."

I spend the day on the phone. Everyone calls—my brother, my niece, my friends of all political persuasions, my reading friends, my writing friends, the brunch club ladies, my friends from the kids' school, and of course, Eloise, Anneke, and Beth. Just like Dickens says: it's the best of times and the worst of times. Billy stops by with a single yellow rose and a plant from Annie. He hugs me with relief and scolds, "You've taken a year off my life!"

We have a wonderful dinner tonight, prepared by Eva from the wine club. They're all taking turns bringing us meals, scheduled and arranged by Carla, who like her hubby Fred, is as conservative and as traditionally religious as they come. Mitch has had his disagreements with her, as have I, but she's as loyal and steadfast as a friend can be.

"I knew you'd be okay. I have faith," Carla says on the phone. I think I have faith now, too, though maybe it's something different than Carla's definition. Maybe I don't believe there's a guy up there sitting on a throne and arranging all the details like a heavenly caterer, but I *do* believe there's a gentle orchestration to life; finding Dr. L with her skilled and caring hands, going for my mammogram when I did, having all this love around me. I do think love and prayers carry weight somehow.

Sometimes this all feels like an exquisite dream—all the love and friendship—and sometimes it feels like a ghastly nightmare. How can life change so much overnight?

Natalie calls to tell me that on the day of my surgery her children's yoga classes and Jill's class all "Om'd" for me. What a charming thought!

I visit Dr. L today for a follow-up exam; it's three days after my surgery. She tenderly examines the site, explaining that the adhesive strips will gradually come loose.

"Everything looks great!" she smiles, but then her tone turns serious. "I won't have the final pathology report until next week, and then we'll know with certainty whether the cancer has infiltrated the nodes."

I sigh with disappointment. More waiting, and just when I thought I had the "all-clear." It's hard to stay in the moment when so much is looming in the future.

Mitch and I take a beautiful walk in the cold sunlight this morning; I step over sticky balls in my path, strewn from the sweet gum trees on the sparkling, frosty sidewalk.

Beth brings a cake over, and Anneke shows up with pizza. Everyone gathers around the dining room table as if we're having a party. Ruthann is in her bliss; there's no New York-style pizza near her home down south.

After my friends leave my sister straightens up while I slip out onto my deck in the night air. I gaze up at the tangled branches of the trees, the blue-gray sky, my small white house, the pictures of my children that rest on a shelf I can glimpse through the window. I think of one word: gratitude.

The day has worn me out, so I hug my sis and head upstairs to bed. As I slip under the covers, I hear the sound of footsteps coming closer in the dark, and two gentle hands reach toward me.

Ben tucks my covers beneath my chin, and kisses me goodnight.

It's a bright mid-January morning, and my sister flies home to North Carolina today; I'm in meltdown mode at the airport. Through my tears, I remind myself of Jill's words: "Everything changes." Ruthann was here for this week, and now she is gone. This is the way things go. I recall the day twenty-two years ago, when she and my mother took the bus to New York City when Aaron was born. I remember hearing their voices outside my hospital room when they first arrived, my tears of relief and joy. When I was a little girl, my sister and I loved one another, but we weren't so close as we are now.

When we arrive home from the airport, I sit at my computer to write; my gaze falls on a picture of my sister and brother and me. It's a photo I had placed in a frame a few months ago, after I came across it in a random box while straightening my home office. I also stumbled upon an empty frame that miraculously fit the photo's two by three inch size so I popped the picture in and put it up on my shelf. In the image, I'm about three years old and Ruthann, then fourteen, stands behind me with her hands on my shoulders. My brother, sixteen, stands next to her, his arms behind him, his feet wide apart. Looking at the picture, I sense that they were protecting me then, just as they are now. (My brother is a private fellow, but let me just say he's been calling me devotedly since my diagnosis.) Who would have thought their baby sister would grow up to have breast cancer, back then, in 1956, when no one even spoke of such things?

The word gratitude comes to mind again. It's strange to be feeling so thankful after finding out one has cancer, but Jill and yoga have taught me how.

This afternoon, I rest in bed, reading a book Ruthann has given me about how water crystals change when they're shown words like "love" and "gratitude." They turn to beautiful shapes after a healing Buddhist prayer, and appear ugly and misshapen when exposed to heavy metal music or harsh words. I race downstairs and write words on paper, taping them to my jar of family tap water: "love, healing, gratitude." The boys look at me with concern, convinced I've gone completely bonkers, but Mitch just shrugs his shoulders. "What have I got to lose?" I grin.

In my wildest dreams I never imagined I'd even jokingly try this sort of thing, or seriously think that any kind of visualization would have a concrete effect. But yoga has changed my outlook; when you open your heart, you also open your mind. There's a lot more in this world that we don't know than we do—I believe that now more than ever— so what the heck.

We meet with the oncologist today. In the waiting area, I overhear a forty-ish woman with three children in tow say she's been coming for treatments for six or seven years. She has her pillow and blanket with her, and a large glass of water with a straw. She sips and lays her head back, then lifts it up to help her boys with their homework, then closes her eyes. "There is one more drug the doctors can try before they run out for good, but only God will make the final decision," she announces.

The place is teeming with people who, I suppose, must have cancer, and I can't believe that I am one of them. I certainly don't *want* to be; I don't want to be like the large, sallow man with swollen fingers and sunken eyes, or the thin bald guy with a beret. I don't want to be among these beautiful young women who probably have breast cancer like me, or to be with these worn out old women, whose expressions are drained and empty.

I rest my head on Mitch's shoulder, and when I'm called in to give blood, tears spring to my eyes. I really don't want to be here at all.

As the technician readies my arm and inserts the needle, I use the "Sa, Ta, Na, Ma" method of self-calming that Natalie has taught me, touching the fingers of my free hand together as I silently repeat the mantra. I don't know why this silly ritual works, but it calms me, and my tears stop.

Next, I'm ushered in to see the oncologist, and Mitch comes along. Dr. B is young, energetic, with a wry sense of humor and a slightly balding head, which probably puts him in league, in one tiny way, with his chemo patients. His touch is gentle, and he makes me laugh. On his desk are pictures of his children, and a row of nuts with silly faces painted on them. Within moments, I'm transformed from a hopeless critic to a hopeful patient. He explains my options clearly and unhurriedly, answering our questions in detail. I'm surprised to learn there's a test that will tell him even more about my particular tumor, and he will use this to determine whether I'll need chemo or not. The only hitch is that the test costs several thousand dollars and may very well not be covered by insurance. It takes us about two seconds to decide to go for it anyway. If there's ever been a time to "splurge" this is it.

On the way out, Mitch asks a nurse if we can peek into the chemo area. "Sure!" she smiles, leading us down a narrow hallway and opening a door to a spacious room. Inside, I see just some men and women in a beauty salon, sitting in chairs watching TV or reading magazines while attendants hover nearby. But that's not quite it, of course. Or is it a beauty salon for the cells? Instead of thinking of this as a poisonous place, I decide to imagine it's a high-tech spa for the cleansing of cancer. I should know by now that you can look at anything from a light or dark perspective. And even though I was reluctant to peer inside that door, I'm grateful that Mitch suggested it. My husband isn't afraid of much, but he believes that when you *are* frightened of something, the best approach is to stare it down (unless, of course, it's a roaming, vicious Rottweiler).

Later in the day, I rest in bed, and gaze out at the sky, totally engrossed in the snarled branches of the tree outside my window. I'm learning to be exactly where I am right now. Still, I think of that woman in the waiting room and how much courage she has. No, I don't want to be part of her world. But since I have no choice in the matter and can't escape, I don't want to be the prisoner who rots in his chains: I want to be the one who writes poetry or finds God.

I'm nervous about testing out this new yoga class tonight, almost as if I'm cheating on Natalie and the Yoga Center, even though she's the one who told me about it. But I'm also anxious to learn what kind of tango yoga and cancer recovery can do together. This is a dance I want to perfect.

So after dinner, I drive the few miles to the new center, and find my way up the stairs to the second-floor studio. Jeanine, a graceful, soft-spoken woman with a twinkle in her deep gray eyes, welcomes me with a strong handshake, and asks me to step into her office to fill out a form. "How are you feeling?" she asks kindly. "Show me how you can move your arm."

I circle widely and she smiles, taking note of my range of motion. "That's wonderful! You're definitely ready for yoga, but just take it slow."

She isn't a youngster though she looks it; sprinkles of silver fleck her curly, blonde hair and her skin is flawless, glowing, and unwrinkled. She's been practicing yoga for thirty-some years.

I'm ushered into the main practice studio, where I place my mat on the floor and choose a blanket and bolster. Even though I'm early, a number of women and a few men are resting on their mats. Music is playing softly and the lights are dim. Even in the low light, I notice that some of these students are my age or older and several are on the hefty side. At last, I've found a yoga class for people of my ilk, after I've already spent a year and a half trying to keep up with Jill and the youthful yogini Mod Squad!

Jeanine leads us in a soft, healing practice, instructing us to yield to our own bodies, letting us take our time with the gentle movements. No one is competing here— if anything, they seem to be holding back. In this "stress and healing" session, we spend a good deal of time reclining, just lazily stretching our toes and our legs. When we finally rise, Jeanine guides us through a very simple series. We bend to the left, then to the right, then forward, our hands behind us in Namaste position. Everything is done slowly and mindfully, and as we move, Jeanine reminds us to be kind to our bodies, to honor ourselves.

I'm feeling so good in this yoga practice that I'm shocked when I find myself in tears in Savasana. Jeanine offers aromatherapy, and as I soothe myself with the drops of jasmine and sandalwood scent, I'm suddenly overcome by grief. How is it possible that I have cancer? It can't be possible that someone who walks for miles, and does yoga, and eats well, and lives happily, can have this disease. The past week flashes through my mind, and I realize how strong I've been, how well I've handled things, how I haven't broken down in front of my children or friends, how much pain and sorrow and fear I've been holding in. Because I'm at yoga, in the dark, on my mat, my feelings come spilling out. I'm quiet in my tears, but they are flowing.

Jeanine uses a healing visualization, and because I'm familiar with this due to Natalie's guidance last week, I know exactly where I'm going. In my mind, I make a beeline for my inner place of comfort, where my "inner healer" resides, and I smell the lilies and lilacs and bask in the cool white light. I feel healing hands on my shoulders, and I know that this is the place I must visit often. I'm grateful that this class has reminded me of where I need to go in my soul.

At the close of the session, I pack up my mat, put away my props, and thank Jeanine, who seems concerned. "Are you okay?" she asks softly, following me to the door, and I nod even though I feel as if I could easily fall to pieces in her arms. I've come on a recommendation from Natalie, after all, and the two are friends. But I know this woman would care about me anyway; yoga practitioners are just that way. I have yet to meet an instructor who doesn't give generously of herself. It seems that the type of people who come to yoga aren't searching for something outside; they're searching for something within, or have already found it and want to help others. The world of yoga is almost like a parallel universe right here on earth, where its inhabitants are peaceful, graceful and kind.

"Healing and stress" yoga is new for me, and I know I'll return to it. Whether it can change anything within the body, I can't prove. But I'm sure it can change my thoughts, and I believe that's half the battle. And anyway, there's a kindness in this yoga center that I want to experience again. I'm learning that kindness toward one's self is yet another reason for practicing yoga. As Jeanine says softly, "Many types of healing can take place on the mat."

∞

I've decided to attend Mitch's concert on this cold, late-January evening. I don't always go to hear him play—it would be impossible to schlep after him everywhere if I wanted a life of my own, and just as unreasonable as expecting him to read every magazine or newspaper piece I've ever written—but when he's performing something special or nearby I do make an effort to be there.

I'm looking forward to this concert, but once here I'm struck by a sense of melancholy. I listen to the music—Handel, Beethoven, and an offbeat piece by Bohuslav Martinu— and wonder what the future holds. If anything, I had thought listening to live classical music would put me in the "now," but my mind is racing, and my thoughts are anything but tranquil.

During the second half of the program, Mitch doesn't perform, so he takes a seat in the empty chair next to me and we hold hands. The next piece is the Brahms Sextet in G Major, Opus 36; all strings. I lay my head on Mitch's shoulder, close my eyes, and my tears fall once again. My gaze rests on Sarah Black, a woman in her sixties, who's playing the violin. She looks so angelic and content; she has a round, cherub face and shiny auburn hair. As she plays her expression is one of pure joy. Such a woman would never get cancer, would only experience the beauty of life; surely Sarah Black has never known the kind of fear that I know now. I'm envious that a woman of her age can play to her heart's content, doing what she loves to do, without fear or worry for her future.

Mitch squeezes my hand and whispers in my ear, not even knowing in the dark where my gaze rests, "Sarah had some kind of cancer about ten years ago. But now she's fine."

I'm overcome with awe and shame.

I play the new Deva Premal tape that my sister has sent me in the mail, and practice yoga at home. I find myself crying during my practice (I guess a side effect of cancer is all these tears! Coupled with the release from yoga, I'm a virtual cascade.) Tomorrow, I plan on going back to Jill's class, but today I'm worrying—not only about whether I'll be able to keep up physically, but whether I'll be able to tolerate it emotionally. I want to be there in that room again so much.

I take a Child's pose, drawing my thoughts inward. I realize what I want is my old life back; the me before the cancer word entered. Would I want to live thirty more years with my eyes closed or three with my eyes open? Frankly, I'd probably pick thirty with eyes shut tight, but in my heart, I know which would be better. I roll up my mat and stand, gazing out at the pear trees.

I just want my carefree existence back. Cancer is the hardest thing I've ever faced—harder than childbirth, harder than my parents' deaths. On Ruthann's advice, I continue to read *The Power of Now*, hanging onto every word like a life jacket. Eckhart Tolle says, "If you have a major illness, use it for enlightenment." Well, I'm sure trying. My past is filled with pain and regret, and also with wonderful experiences that can never be retrieved, and my future is filled with fear and uncertainty. The *now* is a beautiful moment—first stillness, then birds singing as I gaze at the tangle of branches in the sky outside the windows. I don't know why it's so damn hard to be here.

∽

I'm at yoga exactly two weeks after my surgery; Jill and Natalie greet me with hugs and smiles of relief. I can't do my Downward Dog, and I'm really missing it. Funny to think I used to abhor that pose. Jill pays extra attention to me, rubbing my feet, placing her hands on my forehead. I feel like an honored visitor, especially when the woman next to me smiles and whispers, "Welcome back!"

Jill tiptoes from mat to mat during Savasana, but I know she's spending most of her time near me. Still, I can hear her soft footsteps, like those of a visiting nurse going from bed to bed: I've learned the woman to my left is dealing with a serious illness—one of her sons has a rare blood disorder. And across the way is the young woman who will undergo a surgery soon, though the cyst in her breast has been found to be non-cancerous. I'm sure everyone here has a problem, whether small or large. Right now I feel like mine is the worst problem imaginable, but on the other hand, when I think of the woman to my left who is worrying about her child, I know that's not true.

"We are like lotus flowers," Jill says. "We rise from the mud, and bloom into beautiful, white petals, and if it rains, and a drop falls on us, it will simply roll off and away." I like the image of lotus flowers, and decide to incorporate it in my healing vision when I meditate at home. I will picture a vast pond of lotus flowers, all sending out their white light, their goodness, and their strength, their capacity to rise to beauty even in the midst of mud and sorrow.

I attempt Jill's class again today, but the practice is too much for me, and Jill throws me a sideways glance when I try a Downward Dog—as if to warn, "You're not ready yet!" It's almost comical that energetic Jill is trying to slow me down, but I miss my Dog, my Headstand, and everything else. Nevertheless, I content myself with resting on my back and putting my legs "up the wall" when everyone else does inversions. When I started yoga I had to be patient, and patience is called for again.

It's a good lesson to learn because today after class I call the lab in California and discover that my tissue sample for the new test that will help determine my treatment has not arrived. After multiple calls to the lab and my doctor's office, it's revealed that the sample is still hanging out in New Jersey, where it's certainly not supposed to be.

"Damn!" I moan as I hang up. "Now my treatment will be put off even longer! I just want to get started on this."

"Just say Om," Mitch advises, rubbing my neck. "It will be okay."

Tonight, I head out for Jeanine's class. During the meditation/ visualization, she leads us to our "inner healer" or nurturer, and tells us to ask, "Who am I?" This is the same question Jill has asked this morning, instructing us to repeat the question to ourselves over and over for five minutes at the beginning of the class. This morning, I saw a series of images; myself as mother, woman, cancer survivor, and finally, as a child. I felt the most myself when I saw that five-year-old girl, when I realized that so much of me is still just like her. My friend Winston, who lived next door to me when I was young, emailed upon learning that I had cancer, "I knew you before you developed breasts. Are you still that little girl? Are you scared?"

Yes, I am, and tonight during the meditation I can scarcely contain my tears. I am scared as I visit my inner healer, and I still can't believe that I have faced cancer, that this is happening to me.

Both Jeanine and Jill say the same thing: "You are not this body; you are not this mind; you are not your thoughts." Jeanine explains it further: "You are what is divine."

Looking at yoga as a person with a serious disease is different than looking at yoga from the perspective of someone who wants to get in shape or face a few fears that now seem pretty minor when compared to a concrete threat like cancer. I'm *really* searching for answers now, but I'm finding out that they are all inside me.

∞

This morning when I log onto my computer, there's an email from an editor asking me to review a book. I consider whether I should do it for the measly amount it pays, whether I want to spend my time on this sort of work now that I know I have (or have had?) cancer. After a few moments of internal debate, I decide that yes, I do want to keep doing what I've always done, but not at the expense of things I really love, like writing creatively or going to yoga class. But reviewing is fun, and even a meager amount of money is better than none.

The underlying question, then, is do I tell my editor that I had/have breast cancer? Perhaps this will be "too much information." She's asked in her email how I am, so I decide why the hell not. It's not a secret, after all, and I'm finding out that the more I share, the more I learn. Not just about cancer, but about anything. So I type back "Sure! I'd be happy to review the book. As for how I am, I've just had breast cancer surgery, but things are going well."

Within seconds there's a response. Her sister has had breast cancer: a lumpectomy, radiation, then a recurrence, a mastectomy, and chemo. Like a tennis ball, it seems that every time I share my story, a personal story about breast cancer bounces back. This is one hell of a match.

∞

The month of January is almost over; Mitch and I drive to the beach today, even though it's only forty degrees and is supposed to rain. I don't know too many people who would pick up and drive an hour to the beach on a winter morning, but this is one of the advantages of the writer/musician duo, and so we make the most of our unorthodox schedules when we can, whatever the season.

We are here without the kids; they'd all rather sleep in on a Saturday morning. Instead of our children, the piping plovers are scurrying ahead of us, and seagulls dip in and out of the cold waves. The wind is brisk, but with a winter jacket and hat it's bearable. We walk for a half hour and then stop for a hot bowl of chowder at a bar that's just opened. We have the place to ourselves, and for some reason this chowder is the best I've ever eaten; I can detect some kind of alcohol in it, but whether it's wine or whiskey, I can't say.

I'm overwhelmed by my love for my husband, and my desire to spend decades more with him. It's hard to believe that way back when I was wishing he'd take a permanent hike. I can't imagine any man being kinder than he has been to me lately; in the past month, he's bought me six new pairs of shoes! (My close friends call me Imelda because of my infatuation with footwear.) That's just silliness, I know, but this effort to bring me to the beach, to feed me well, to listen to my fears and worries…I'm ashamed that I ever caused him a moment's pain.

On our walk back, we pass by the plovers again, the fishermen, the gulls, the bits of sea glass and one lone horseshoe crab. Suddenly, along the dunes I spot a flash of red. I grab Mitch's arm and we stand motionless, watching a huge red fox racing through the brush. What a glorious vision! I admire the way he travels, as if he's totally in the moment and loving his life.

"Want to stop for pizza?" Mitch inquires on the way home.

"You need to *ask?*" I smile. The first summer we dated, Mitch and I went on a mission to sample every pizza within a twenty-mile radius of our hometown. I suspect that the clincher in our love affair was my impressive ability to handily devour four slices.

We pull into a place we visit only when we're "down the shore" and order two decafs first to warm up. The waiter keeps filling Mitch's coffee cup, and I'm struck by how this simple act eases my heart; the small things that certain people do can make a huge difference in how we remember a day.

We're back home in time to fix dinner for the kids; while I'm heating up the water for pasta, I pop into my office to check my email. (Virginia Woolf might be pleased that I have a writing room of my own but I wonder what she'd think of its close proximity to my kitchen.) I'm surprised to find a message from a woman in town who had breast cancer ten years ago. We're just acquaintances, but now that she's reached out to me (hearing about my plight through our small town's phenomenal rumor hotline), I know that we'll have a deeper connection. It's funny, because I've thought of her often in the past month. I try to envision strong, surviving women whenever I can.

It's Sunday; Jill picks me up and we drive to another yoga center where she also teaches to listen to a young Tibetan monk speak. The studio is crowded with yoginis on bolsters, excitedly awaiting the arrival of the guru guest. Within moments he enters, looking— to me, anyway— like a Rutgers student dressed in a toga. He begins to talk about…well, I honestly don't know what the hell he's talking about. And turns out he *is* originally from Jersey.

I squirm on my mat, glancing around the room; behind me is a guy sitting peacefully, twirling in his hand a beautiful golden thread. I nudge Jill quietly and she whispers, "Tibetan prayer wheel." I've never heard of such a thing before, and I'm tempted to stare like a tourist in New York City. I guess even Buddhists have their sacred toys.

Two hours later, the monk rises and bids us farewell. I don't want to insult Jill, but on the way out I ask, "Did you enjoy the lecture? I found it hard to follow."

"It *was* a bit convoluted," she admits.

Still, it's been fun to "hang out." I can't imagine going to hear a Tibetan monk with most of my other girlfriends, though Eloise would probably dig it. It seems strange to use the word girlfriend with Jill, but I do feel that she's much more to me than just a yoga teacher now. She's more like an angel who was sent to help me through this time in life, but I'm also quite sure we're going to remain friends forever.

This entire experience reminds me of the fact that I actually have a Buddha sitting in my living room. The two-foot high statue is in a glass cupboard that I never open; Mitch's uncle, a wealthy, generous man who travels widely, gave it to us about fifteen years ago. After Jill drops me home I open the case and stare at the figure inside. His arms are bent at the elbows, and the hands are stretched upwards and toward me, as if in a gesture of protection.

I hold the glass door to the case ajar and stare into the Buddha's solemn eyes. "Are you doing your job?" I demand. "Or have you kacked out on me?"

Healing Hands

In class today, we imagine the colors of our "chakras," which are—according to Eastern wisdom—invisible energy centers or "wheels" found in the body. I'm partial to the last one—which apparently is situated at the top of the head: white light. I've been envisioning white light for the past few months, ever since my diagnosis. I know the research says that meditation and visualization help somehow, and I wonder whether Wendy Wasserstein, who died yesterday of lymphoma, tried them. When someone dies of cancer, everyone in the cancer community must inhale sharply. I did, anyway.

Class is quiet today, and I keep up with it fairly well, returning tentatively to my Downward Dog. I don't want to push too much, and I try to remember the patience word.

After class I call my oncologist, Dr. B, to check on the status of the test that we're waiting on. They *still* haven't sent my tissue sample to the lab, so Mitch and I head over in person to sign the form again and straighten out the delay. This time I'm not as intimidated by the office; I see the cancer patients and I know that I'm one of them. I'm "in the club" as we used to say in high school (though this is one club I'd sure like to quit!).

∞

Since it's Groundhog Day—a day I've always found to be amusing and propitious—I check my horoscope online and discover I'm going to face a bump in the road, but I'll "learn from the experience." My cousin has called this a "bump in the road," too, and I can only wish that he and this cyber-psychic were right. It feels a lot bigger than a bump to me. Tooling around this website, I come across a lot of other fascinating items; meditation circles, communicating with angels, divining...all kinds of wacko stuff. I wonder why so many people seem to be returning to the Middle Ages. Maybe it's because our contemporary world has gone, as my kids always say, "mad-crazy."

How fitting that we do a "walking meditation" in yoga class today, a practice we've never tried before. We walk in silence in an oval shape for about ten minutes, pausing between steps. I'm thinking mostly about the pert little feet of the woman ahead of me, but now and then my mind completely empties. The process is soothing, and I notice that as we walk our oval draws smaller and smaller. We seem to find comfort in drawing together as we move.

After class, I open the glass case and stare some more at my Buddha, contemplating what his hand gesture means. I'm pretty sure it's a young male, but it could be female. I like the way his hands are positioned; I do hope he is protecting me. I hope he's protecting all of us.

∞

Today, while taking Sam to the dermatologist, I happen

upon a wonderful article about breast cancer in a magazine that someone has left on a chair in the waiting room. I pick it up by chance as I was intending to read a book I've brought along. But there it is, full of fascinating material about things like green tea and turmeric (both are cancer fighters), just seemingly waiting for me. Who left it there and why? I consider stealing the magazine, but write down the website address instead to print out online. Maybe another woman will come to have her kid's wart removed and learn about breast cancer, too.

My book group meets tonight at a bar in the swanky nearby town where they all live, the same town where my writer friends reside. I've heard from everyone in the group, but this is the first time most are seeing me since my surgery. I'm sort of wondering if they'll expect me to *look* different, and I've tried my best with my hair, makeup, and clothing tonight. I don't want to appear to be the worried mom that I am.

To my surprise, all the ladies think I look grand. I don't *feel* very grand, and I'm still scared as hell. But it's nice to be with my girlfriends and to drink one glass of red wine. We scarcely talk about the book we've read; *Teacher Man* by Frank McCourt, though many of us like it. We talk instead about our children. It's funny how women so often run away from their families for an evening, and then spend the whole time chatting about their kids.

I've been avoiding writing today, avoiding just about everything. For some reason I feel more hopeless and down than I felt just two weeks ago.

I go to yoga, though I don't really want to. Before class, the student who led me through those strange energy exercises a while ago approaches and grabs my hand. "How are you doing?" she asks eagerly.

"I'm in waiting mode. Just waiting for the results of that lab test, waiting to see what my treatment will be."

"Don't wait for life to happen," she advises, shaking her head. "Life is happening *now.*"

I'm grateful to hear these words. There are so many wise women at yoga.

Jill talks about bumblebees, how they hum, take what they need from a flower without harming it, how they're busy and focused, how they shouldn't really be able to fly, given their shape, but this fact doesn't prevent them; they just fly anyway. I've often thought we all *sound* like bumblebees when we Om, but maybe we're like them in other ways, too, just forging ahead with our lives, doing what we know we must do.

Because of my bladder problems—not to reveal *all* my gory health issues, but I seem to live in the bathroom lately—I visit a urologist my internist has recommended. He seems like a pleasant man—but when he tells me he'll need to do a cystoscopy (an uncomfortable procedure to take a "look-see" inside and determine that there are no cancerous polyps) I panic. "It's a lot to handle, with the breast cancer and all."

He looks me straight in the eye. "But you're handling it well, aren't you? You *are* handling it."

Something about the way he speaks seems unusually personal for a physician. He feels almost like a friend, and so I offer, "It's okay. I'll use my yoga breathing."

"*I* do yoga," the doctor says.

I'm so surprised. We laugh and talk about yoga, and it turns out he knows Jill. He knows my wonderful teacher!

"You're going to be okay," the doctor says, and for some reason, I feel calmer. As I leave, we bow to one another and say "Namaste." Now, *that's* my kind of doc.

I scurry to my car, realizing I have just enough time to make it to my next appointment with my ob/gyn (it turns out *she* does gyrokinesis, whatever that may be!) As long as I'm frequenting doctors, what's one more, and anyway I'm due for a checkup. I tell her about my bladder and she orders a sonogram (of course, by now it's occurred to me that maybe it's ovarian cancer that's the problem). The more doctors, the more tests; the more symptoms, the more fears. In the past, it was easy to brush off an ache or pain as something trivial since I'd been so healthy all my life. But now I'm a cancer survivor, and even though breast cancer didn't cause me any pain, if I'd been paying closer attention to my body I might have found that lump earlier.

I wonder if there will be a time when all this will be over, a happy time, that is. I've heard others say that once you start on the doctor treadmill, it's hard to ever get off. I'd like to be on my yoga mat, not on this path.

"Is there something else that's bothering you?" my ob/gyn asks. She's a very intuitive lady.

I clear my throat. "Well, there's this little thing called sex. I haven't really felt like doing it since my surgery, and I just can't face using my diaphragm any more. Anyway, my periods have been fading for a year or more. Menopause is definitely catching up with me."

My doctor looks at my chart, smiles and suggests, "Get yourself some personal lubricant and go to town!" Finally, I'm too old to get pregnant!

This long day of appointments has tired me out, but I decide the best antidote is Jeanine's class, where I bask in the beauty of her gentle voice. During Savasana, in the darkened room with the candles lit, Jeanine talks about grieving. "We can grieve for a person we've lost, but also for a part of ourselves. We can grieve for the loss of our health or the loss of a part of our bodies. We can grieve for a wounded part of our soul," she says.

We're to put our hand over our heart and feel it beating, but mine lands on my breast. I hold it there, thinking that it's not that little bit of flesh that I miss, but the idea that I was so healthy and strong.

"Remember," Jeanine whispers into the darkness, "all healing takes time."

∞

The oncologist's office calls. Dr. B says I have scored low on the Oncotype DX test, which means I may not need chemo! Studies have actually shown that in some cases, (and I seem to be one of them) chemo may actually be "overkill."

To celebrate, Mitch and I purchase some new silky brand of KY jelly, lingering in front of the counter at the grocery store like teenagers buying their first condoms. We don't know that vaginal lubricant comes in "hot" or thermal, or that you can now buy rubbers in pretty, feminine packaging. We haven't shopped for this kind of stuff in thirty years. That's how long I've been using that damned diaphragm.

The young pharmacist sits frowning behind a glass window, probably wondering why we old fogies are ogling the contraceptives. I find a jar of duck sauce on a shelf nearby and place it in between the tubes of KY. "Works just as well," I giggle to Mitch as we head home to try our new product.

Later in the afternoon, I email my friends to tell them about my test results. Billy calls me as soon as he gets my message. "You see," he says, "it's the power of prayer. We're gonna turn you into a church-goer, yet!"

I don't think that's going to happen. But I don't believe it's just coincidence that my urologist practices yoga, or that I find a magazine with a wonderful article on breast cancer on the chair next to me when I take Sam to the dermatologist to get his wart removed.

I remember the little girl with the bluebird picture we once found in Cape May —the same print I had on my wall as a child, the same picture that Ruthann and my brother and I all wanted when my mother died because as kids we all thought that little girl was our mom (my brother got to keep it, because he asked for so little). Why did I find that picture in the bathroom of a bed and breakfast? (The owner sold it to me for a song.)

Why *anything*, indeed? If you start asking that question the fact that there *is* an answer eventually becomes obvious. Like Billy says, if only because there *has* to be.

Before bed, I read that one of the paths to "awakening" is through a serious illness or a traumatic event. The book also says that awakening doesn't happen all at once—it's a lengthy process.

I remember something that Ali once said: "We, too, can be Buddhas. We, too, can be awake."

This is one hell of an alarm clock.

On this drizzly February Saturday evening, I pick up Anneke; we drive to Comedy Night—a fundraiser for Sam's graduating class. We sit at a table with my wine club friends, and I sip my one glass of red wine (which I probably shouldn't even be having) as they throw back volumes. I wonder if I'll ever get drunk again. I wonder, too, if my decision not to drink much of anything anymore will limit my ability to tolerate Republicans.

I chat with Robin (one of the few liberals in our group) about yoga. She brings it up, because she knows my practice must be helping me through this time. "I can't imagine going through something like cancer. I love life; life is awesome," Robin sighs.

One of the moms at the event is pouting because I didn't tell her about my dilemma. Now that she knows, thanks again to the rumor hotline, she says she'll add me to her prayer list. I imagine that quite a few people in the room know about my cancer, but they're keeping mum. This is Comedy Night, after all, and the comedians are telling jokes. They even tell a few about death, which I don't find very funny.

But that's all right; my conservative friend Fred is offended by the jokes about Condi Rice. And there's a prissy mom across the room who scowls whenever there's a joke about blowjobs. This guy is good; he has something offensive for everyone. Still, I'm relieved when the event is over; I drop Anneke at her door and head home.

Snow falls heavily in the night, and when I awaken and look outside the sparrows on the tops of the hedges resemble figures in Japanese ink drawings. I watch from my upstairs windows as they gather at my feeder, pecking frantically, as if they've been starved for days, though my feeder is always full for them. One sparrow is on my deck, hopping around in the pocket of safety beneath a chair. Then he hops out into the snow and back again, ruffling his feathers. I've never noticed so many birds out playing in the snow before. But maybe I just haven't ever *really* looked.

Life *is* awesome, as Robin says.

∞

In the fresh snow, Mitch and I slog to town and have lunch at the diner, which is the only restaurant open. The trees are covered with thick flakes, and the walking is tough, but we manage.

After our walk, we shop for dinner. I think of the meatballs and chicken (no doubt pumped with hormones) I passed up at Comedy Night, and I purchase some seaweed salad. My diet has changed; I'm buying everything organic and taking supplements by the truckload— turmeric, green tea capsules, garlic. I'm following the advice of anyone with an opinion—the librarian who says to eat blueberries, my mother-in-law, who says to take maitake mushroom. I want to be here for a very long time.

The kids are happy to be snowed in, and they invite some friends over. I realize that of the eight boys who are here, two in addition to mine have mothers who have had breast cancer. I know these women well enough; they didn't smoke, or drink too much or gorge on red meat. I wonder what's going on in this country. Talk about conspiracy theories!

Eloise calls tonight and we have a long chat about my ailments—she listens to every detail, just as my mother might. I've figured out what it is that Eloise gives me: pure sympathy and love, straight up, unwavering and strong, like a dry martini. The difference between Eloise and my mom, however, is that if she's worried, Eloise doesn't show it, and when I go down a morbid trail, she gently takes my hand and leads me back.

Not that anyone would want to know this, but my poop was bright red today, and the water in the toilet was the color of blood. All day, I'm convinced that I have colon cancer.

When I confess this to Eloise she asks, "Have you been eating beets?"

"Shit, yes! Organic ones."

"So much for health food!" Eloise laughs.

Thank God I'm back at yoga. I missed last Thursday, and I feel like it's been forever.

Jill says she's been thinking about the word "already," and she tells us that no matter what we're going through we've "already" been here before. I have to mull this one over, and I don't know if I agree with her. I've never been through anything like this; I've never had to dig this deep to find the strength to face a challenge.

In Savasana, though, I recall the days on which my parents died, and I remember how deeply I had to search for the strength to get through their funerals. Learning that you have cancer seems totally different. But maybe it isn't. I realize I have "already" had to face terrible waves of fear in my life; in fact, maybe all those rehearsals were just warm-ups for the biggest fear of all: confronting my own mortality. Facing cancer, after all, is in some ways even worse than facing death. If you're going to die—in many cases—you don't even know it. You're plowed down by a crazy driver, or suddenly stricken with a heart attack. But cancer gives you time to cozy up to the idea. You can mull over all the things you've done right or wrong in your life; you have the time while undergoing chemo or other treatments to decide whether you want to be bitter and angry, or grateful for what you've had.

When Sam was a toddler, he once wandered out of the house. For ten minutes, we couldn't find him. I think of where my heart and mind went on that day when Mitch and I were frantically racing up and down our street, searching and calling his name. I remember that dreamy sense of running but feeling that my legs weren't moving, my heart thumping high in my chest. I remember feeling as if the world was ending within my own body, the sensation that nothing could ever, ever be right again, the overwhelming fear that he'd been kidnapped, or hit by a car, or drowned in a neighbor's swimming pool. (Sam, clad only in his diaper, eventually showed up in the backyard, blissfully pushing his plastic toy bubble lawnmower.)

Remembering those moments, I realize I have "already" been to some very scary places in my life, and somehow, I did find the strength to put one foot in front of the other, to follow one heartbeat with the next. I think we've all had moments like these, and yes, we've "already" been there. We've all had moments when we thought we couldn't make it to the other side of a lake, or we couldn't get around that huge truck headed straight at us. Those fears are everywhere (and the realities, too). Everyone faces them, and sometimes the fear is even worse than the real outcome, though we suffer either way. We suffer even when we don't need to suffer. And then, when we realize that suffering and worrying won't get us anywhere, we find strength.

After yoga Mitch and I drive to a popular Spanish restaurant for a Valentine's Day lunch. Our plates are heaped with veggies, fish and other healthy foods. To look at us, no one would know we've been married for twenty-eight years; we're having so much fun. And yet, if this cancer thing hadn't come into our lives, I bet we'd be complaining or I'd be aggravated with him. Because of it, we're laughing and eating, and making the most of our time together. I remember one of our very first dates; we'd gone to a local ice cream shop and ordered two cold drinks called "Fribbles." As soon as we put in our order the absurdity of the word struck us both at exactly the same moment. We spent the next half hour laughing our asses off; in fact, we were laughing and snorting so fiercely that we could scarcely swallow our Fribbles when they arrived. I knew in a flash this was a guy I could really love.

On days like today, it's hard to believe that there were years when Mitch and I argued constantly, years when the weight of three small children and two burgeoning careers was more than we could manage. But today, those arguments are long past, and even our disappointments—the times when my manuscripts were rejected, or when Mitch failed to win an audition even though he'd practiced so hard—seem not so horrid, and at least we had each others' arms to fall into. We're here, after all, together. I always thought it totally unnecessary for bad things to happen to appreciate what we have; but the truth is, we do sometimes need to step into the darkness to understand how bright our light really is.

After lunch, we set out for yet another test—I have my ultrasound today, at the suggestion of my ob/gyn, who is following up on my bladder discomfort. Mitch comes into the examining room with me and watches with fascination as the technician gently pokes the tip of a long dildo type instrument up my crotch and peers around inside. The picture on the screen intrigues my husband, but I'm too nervous to look. Instead, I search the technician's face for hints that something is wrong.

On the way out, the technician calls out, "Don't you worry, hon! Things seem to be just fine."

We thank her for the thumbs up and then skip to the car like six-year-olds.

When we get home Mitch suggests we have sex to celebrate… but I tell him I've already had some today.

I talk to Eloise tonight for a long time on the phone, and we laugh and laugh. "I've read that cancer loves sugar," I say.

"Why can't cancer love rutabagas? Why can't it love broccoli rabe?" Eloise jokes, but then she turns serious. "I don't want to bring up the topic of cancer unless *you* say you want to talk about it. That's what my sister's friend who had breast cancer suggests."

"You can broach the topic any time," I explain, "but what I *really* don't like is when people bring it up when I'm in the middle of a joke. I'm just at the punch line and they butt in with, 'And how do you feel about your cancer?' That's what your sister's friend means."

∞

I wonder if I'm OD-ing on yoga. I go this morning to Jill's class and tonight I plan to hit Jeanine's. The two are so different. I do a Headstand today—just for a few seconds. It feels so good to get back up there! I'm up and down so swiftly that Jill doesn't even see me. I'm actually afraid she'll tell me to slow down!

I have something to cheer about today. After class, Mitch and I see Dr. B and he proclaims that I can definitely forgo chemo and skip directly to radiation. I never thought I'd see a day when I was jubilant to get to radiation, but here it is. I will also take a hormone therapy pill for the next five years because my cancer was estrogen-receptor positive, which basically means it thrived on estrogen, so now we're going to deprive it of its favorite snack.

Before dinner, I take a walk alone while Mitch retreats to our bedroom to practice his clarinet. It's cold and bright out, and as I'm striding up the avenue, I nearly turn my ankle on a couple of those sticky balls that fall from the sweet gum tree. I gaze down at those damn balls scattered all over the place. Yes, sometimes you stumble on them, and some you avoid altogether. And some you just kick the fuck out of your way.

In the morning, my ob/gyn calls to say my ultrasound is normal. I have ovaries, I have a bladder, and they look dandy. I hope I can put some of my fears to rest now, though I know that being dealt the cancer card once in life is going to make me wary that I'll draw that hand again.

Anneke sweeps in tonight with her wine, a fresh bag of decaf coffee beans, and some pistachio nuts. We talk about friends from our past—she's been dreaming about some of hers, and she wants to reconnect. I think of the many people I've been in contact with in the past few months. It's not as though I'd ever lost communication with them, but having cancer has put everyone on alert. My inbox is full each morning, and my phone still rings often. Just today I received an email from a woman I met five years ago while camping in Vermont. We've exchanged cards every Christmas, and this year I sent her a note in January, just catching up. Today she reveals that she went through chemo when she was in her early thirties. When you share your own losses and fears others open up and share theirs. Everyone has them. Yes, everyone.

Today, Jill's subject is desires— we're not supposed to go

overboard. But isn't it okay to desire health, or happiness, or love? I guess as long as you don't go around shooting people to get these things. I don't really have any desires lately other than to get my health back and live a long life. The things I wanted before—a new kitchen, a bigger house, a nicer car—seem really lame now.

Jill demonstrates the amazing King Pigeon pose today, managing to hold both hands behind her head while grabbing onto her ankle. She's quite a contortionist, but she admits it took her five years to achieve this particular asana. Her muscles bulge and her curly red hair shimmers as she arches into the pose. I'm quite content with reaching behind my back with one hand. I'm quite content just to be here.

After class, I walk to town to get a haircut. I've been putting this off, waiting to see if I will have any hair to cut. Now that I know I'm going to do radiation without chemo, I'm due for a trim. Still, I feel guilty, thinking about the cancer victims (are we victims?) who will lose their hair during treatment. I think about how I've admired my long hair lately; once I agreed to grow it, I really liked it, and I'd spend time in front of the mirror brushing and styling. When I got my diagnosis it actually crossed my mind that God was punishing me for my vanity and would now take away my hair (well, I was raised in a Christian church, and in spite of the kindness of Jesus there's a lot of sinner and vengeance stuff in the Bible that's hard to shake). But it turns out that wasn't true. Maybe, however, we are all meant to think about why we spend so much time preening our bodies when we really should be preening our souls.

Or, maybe I just need to be thinking about why I insisted on keeping my hair short for so long, even though Mitch prefers it long. It's a control issue, I'm sure, and I do like to have control of my own body. On the other hand, I've been known to walk up to his ponytail with a pair of scissors and just snip off a few inches. He's not happy about that because for some odd reason he thinks his long hair helps get him gigs: "Hire whatshisname... you know, the guy with the long gray ponytail."

When I sit in my hairdresser's chair and announce, "I'm not going to need chemo!" she throws her arms around me. It's not just because she's happy she'll still have me as a customer. Irene's been cutting my hair since before she had kids—at least ten years. She's part of my life and I'm part of hers, and that in itself is a reason to throw our arms around each other.

The trim she gives me today is perfectly tapered and shaped; she takes her time, and her fingers feel light and gentle. At the finish, she holds the mirror up for me to inspect; this, indeed, is the most beautiful haircut I've ever received. Everyone gives what he or she can, but the source is always the same: love.

Mitch and I stop at a nutrition center today so that he can buy some Pycnogenol, which is supposed to help your heart (it's also supposed to help your dick, we've heard). I've been taking all kinds of supplements in addition to my cancer chasing hormone therapy pill. Turmeric, green tea extract, garlic pills, selenium, a host of supplements I've found in various books. Today, I'm not shopping for anything in particular, but I'm mesmerized by all the choices. Dandelion, celery, red wine extract (why not just drink a bottle of good Merlot?), CoQ10, grape seed, and Gotu Kola. The choices are endless. If someone took all of these things, would they kill themselves or live forever?

I was raised on *Coca* Cola and white bread. Sure, there were health food stores back in the Fifties (my piano teacher ate seaweed and believed in spirits, so I know New Agers existed, even then). But most of us were oblivious; salt, sugar and butter flowed in my house like manna. My mother just sent me to the door when the Freihofer man arrived with his horse and cart—

the bakery's quaint tradition in our upstate town—and told me to pick out whatever I pleased. Usually, I selected cream-filled cupcakes or raspberry pie. My mother didn't blink an eye, and often offered a soda to go with my snack, since sugar had not yet been demonized.

What a different world I live in today. It's good to see that so many people are becoming aware of what's in –and not in—our food supply. But I'm concerned about the many others who will get sick before they wake up. And no one knows, really, what causes one person to succumb to an illness or not.

Mitch comes up from behind, gives me a nudge, and pulls me out of the store. I could stand here all day, just wondering which bottle holds the magic bullet.

Jill hugs me today, and apologizes for something she said in class last week, that we "get what we deserve." She hopes I didn't take it the wrong way.

It's funny, because I *did* think about those words, but not in the way I would have in the past. I don't believe I "deserved" to have cancer, or that anyone does.

But I do deserve to learn how essential it is to be where I am, and not to let my thoughts continually wander into the past and future. I do deserve to learn how much my friends and family mean to me, and how much I mean to them. I do deserve to realize how much yoga has changed my life. These things I do deserve. I know that's what Jill has meant, and that's exactly the way I take it.

Tonight, at Jeanine's class, I let myself think about my mother. I envision a picture of her that I keep on my piano; she's smiling, with her arms crossed behind her head, her elbows lifted. The photo was taken a few years after my father died, on a trip to the seashore; Mitch's mom had rented a cottage and we had all gone for a few days. I think that weekend was the first time Mom realized she was going to be able to go on with her life without Dad; it was okay to smile again, and enjoy her grandchildren. Until now, when I've thought of my mother, I've been in her last week of life, when she was afraid and in pain. I'm going to try to keep that other, happy picture in my mind.

Jeanine leads us in a swaying Palm Tree pose. "Like the tree, we too can bend and sway and be buffeted by winds," she reminds us, "but if our roots are deep we will stay standing. We will stay strong."

∞

Gino is visiting Sam today. He shyly approaches me in the living room and asks softly, "How *are* you?"

"I feel good," I answer, meeting his deep brown eyes. We're talking now as two cancer survivors, not as a boy and the mom who has known him since Kindergarten.

"How are your treatments going?"

"I'll be doing radiation," I respond, knowing he went through a full round of chemo. "I don't know how you did it, but you're my inspiration."

"You do what you have to do," Gino smiles. He is a seventeen-year-old with a grown man's wisdom.

My own children don't ask me how I'm doing, how I'm feeling; I don't think they want to know—God forbid I should say I'm doing badly. They *have* noticed that I'm in bed each night by ten; I want to get a good night's rest, and I've read that early to bed, early to rise really is healthier than staying up till all hours of the night ranting along with liberal talk radio. I've read, too, that research suggests women who get cancer have spent their lives putting others first. I imagine this is true. I do feel it's time for me to take care of myself. In the past, I might flee my family to drink too much wine with my girlfriends. Now I'm fleeing them for sleep, for yoga, for long walks.

Still, sometimes I worry that I'm letting them down, especially Ben, who's spending even more time on the computer, even more time with friends, which I suppose is what he'd be doing anyway. I worry that I'm neglecting him, though his grades are great and he seems happy. He's always been an easy child, but now I wonder how easy things have really been for *him* lately. When I ask if he wants to talk about my illness, he declines. When I ask if he has told his friends, he says no. Yet, he lets me know when they discuss mammograms in science class, and he's curious about what goes on at my doctor's visits. He's fourteen and a boy, after all, so I don't really expect much chitchat. He still lets me hug him, though; all my children do.

Once when Sam was heading off to Cub Scout camp for a week, at the bus the first day, one mom warned me, "Now, don't go hugging him in front of everyone, you'll embarrass him." Just then, Sam broke away from the line and ran straight at me, throwing his arms around my neck, proclaiming loudly, "I love you, Mom!"

I don't want my boys to be embarrassed by love. So far, it looks like they've learned this lesson.

∞

It's late February, still frigid cold, but we take a family hike, which is no mean feat because now that our children are twenty-two, seventeen, and fourteen you can bet no one wants to be with their parents at 9 o'clock on a weekend morning. Nevertheless, this is something Mitch wants to do, so we've all agreed to go along with it.

Deep in the woods the wind isn't too strong and the kids seem almost happy to be here. They're frolicking like toddlers, and I'm almost just as nervous as when they *were* toddlers because the trail has suddenly veered perilously close to the edge of an enormous cliff. Overlooking the depths of the Hudson River, I'm suddenly paralyzed by fear. Mitch and the boys have bounded ahead by now, leaving me—the fifty-three-year-old cancer survivor—behind. As I stand frozen in place, I suddenly realize how this whole scene fits into my life. The kids and Mitch are racing ahead, thrashing through life, healthy and unafraid, while I'm here on my breast cancer journey, terrified, immobile and alone. It doesn't help to see the face of death so up close again, either; one wrong step and I could easily plunge five hundred feet into the frigid water.

I angrily force myself down a few more steps, but then I call out to Mitch that if he doesn't get his ass back here *right now* I am really going to lose it. The urgency in my voice catches his attention; he turns around and scrambles back up the trail. "What's the matter?" he asks, in that innocent puppy dog tone that men use when they know they've done something really idiotic.

I don't want my boys to see me acting like a baby, so I turn my head to hide my tears. I know I'm crying a lot lately, and really I'm not always so emotional, but it hasn't even been two months since my surgery, and I have radiation yet to endure. Perhaps I'm just a tad bit fragile still.

We head back to the car and drive home, everyone but me seemingly thrilled that we all had a near-death experience as a family.

Later in the day, I have a colossal fight with Mitch, the first we've had in months. "You should go back to the therapist," he snaps. "Obviously, yoga isn't working."

I don't have the energy to argue, and maybe he's right; this whole yoga thing is malarkey. I was definitely not acting strong, or using my breathing, or being in the now today. I was just like my old self, standing on a cliff, imagining that my children, my husband and I would all go crashing over.

I attend a lecture on Patanjali's sutras at Jeanine's yoga center tonight (these are sort of like the Ten Commandments for the yogic world, though there are 196 of them, which is a hell of a lot more than ten). The older woman who is teaching the class is very kind, but she's not making the sutras very clear. I'm still figuring out what the word karma really means, and now she's throwing all kinds of other Indian phrases around: niyama, yama, Minnehaha, whatever. Apparently all these asanas I've been doing for the past year and a half are just the tip of the yogic iceberg. This yogini says that the asanas are really just the "preparation" for meditation, so I guess I've been twisting myself silly for eighteen months just so I can close my eyes and do some non-thinking.

To wit, we meditate. I have no idea what to meditate about— or if one is even supposed to meditate *about* anything— but since the teacher has mentioned the word "journey" I take that as a cue, and within moments I'm on that cliff again. It wasn't just the five hundred foot plunge into the freezing cold river that so frightened me, it was the idea that I was being left behind, left alone to face my own journey, my own battle with cancer.

I've always been afraid of being alone, even though I love solitude. But the solitude I love isn't limitless; an hour to sip tea and read a novel is not the same as a one-on-one with eternity. Having a disease makes you realize that we really *are* alone, you can't really share the pain and fear of an illness with anyone, and that's why it's so essential to learn how to reach inside for strength. I don't know why I tried to chase after my boys on that cliff anyway. If I'd just waited quietly alone in the woods until their return, I'd have been where *I* needed to be. I'd have respected my own pace, my own body and soul.

For the first time in months, I awaken in the night with my hands clenched into fists. Where are my Namaste hands? Where is my calming prayer position?

∞

Before class this morning I tell Jill about my cliff experience. "We all have moments like that," Jill says, "and look at all you're dealing with." I've forgotten that yoga is about forgiveness and acceptance as well as about being strong. Maybe it's okay to have a meltdown now and then, and maybe by the edge of a five hundred foot drop into the frigid Hudson River is a perfectly acceptable place to do that. I'll try to get back up on my "mountain," to find my Tadasana, but I'm not going to beat myself up for a moment of weakness. I'm not going to assume that because yoga didn't work "at that moment" that yoga doesn't work. It's not a question of "working," anyway. Yoga is not a magic bullet any more than a health supplement is.

After we "Om," Jill refers to her lesson of the other day, in which she said we get what we deserve. She modifies her message, explaining that what she really believes is, "We get what we need." If we need to be awakened, something will open our eyes.

CHAPTER TWENTY-TWO: MARCH

The Radiance of Being Radiated

A new month. Jill discusses the asanas today, but she also reminds us that there are actually seven *other* limbs of yoga (ethical principles, rules of personal conduct, breathing techniques, control of the senses, concentration of the mind, meditation, and union with the divine). Jill thinks you can get to most of them by doing the asanas, but some yogis apparently believe the asanas shouldn't come first. This is all too confusing for me. Still, I think I do know the most important thing: just keep practicing.

I'm beginning to worry about my meeting with the radiation oncologist, which is scheduled for Monday. The past few days, I've been thinking less and less about cancer. Now I'll have to face the topic head-on again. I take a nice long walk today in the sunny cold weather. As I pass a tall sycamore tree along my chosen path, a cacophony of crows sings out. It's amazing how hundreds of birds can fit in one tree, and I wonder why they've chosen this particular tree for their congregation. Just as weird is the fact that when I pass by on my way home, not a single crow is left.

"We are all neck-deep in grace," writes the Buddhist philosopher/psychologist Jack Kornfield.

Anneke comes by tonight, and we talk about her new passion: voice lessons! "This has changed my life!" she exclaims happily. "My teacher is a gem. She's only about thirty, with big blue eyes and long blonde hair. She has so much knowledge, a beautiful voice, and such patience!"

I'm reminded of Jill, and I'm so thrilled that Anneke, too, has discovered that even in middle age you can learn something new. It's wonderful that we can learn from younger women, just as they can learn from us.

Just before bed, I check my email and find a reassuring message from a dear fellow writer from my magazine days: "You were always radiant, so now, for a little while, you'll be radiated." I'll try to keep that sentiment in mind.

It's the first Sunday of the month, and I attend a free meditation circle that's starting tonight at Jeanine's. I figure anything that calms my mind is a valid activity (short of drugs and alcohol). We all sit on mats or blankets and Jeanine says she will "ring" us in.

"Just follow your breath," Jeanine instructs, as she taps her little portable chime, and we close our eyes. I squint mine open to spy what the others are doing, and sure enough, no one's doing anything at all. We're a group of twenty women ages twenty-five to seventy, sitting silently with our eyes closed as if we have time to kill.

Within a few moments, my thoughts turn to an annoying pain up my spine, a recurring itch on my left nostril, and the sensation of having to swallow. I'm not sure what purpose this will serve if all I do is sit here thinking about itches and cramps and wishing it were over.

The second part of the session is a walking meditation. This time, we walk back and forth across the room, staggering our paths so that we don't bump into one another. I wonder what people rushing by in their cars outside the window might be thinking when they see two dozen women slowly walking back and forth as if in a hypnotic trance. Most likely, they think we've downed some electric Kool-Aid and we're headed for Comet Hale-Bopp. That's what I might figure had I driven by this place a year ago.

But not any more. Now I know we're a bunch of women who need to calm our hearts and minds.

The dreaded March 6 meeting day has arrived, but I'm surprisingly calm. Maybe this has something to do with the meditation. More likely it's just that the *anticipation* of many of these meetings and procedures is far worse than the meetings and procedures will really be. Mitch and I sit in comfy couches in the waiting room, next to a TV where Rachael Ray is stirring up a mouth-watering sauce. I'm tempted to whip out my notebook and jot down the recipe, but my name is called. Apparently, radiation therapy runs on a highly efficient timetable.

Dr. G is sweet and tiny, with a hearty laugh. She has round, black-rimmed glasses and she wears her hair in a girlish ponytail. Dr. G explains the process and purpose of the radiation, answering Mitch's many questions. She assures us that they'll do their best to accommodate *my* schedule, even when Mitch jokes that my primary concern is getting to yoga class.

"We don't want to disrupt your life, and we certainly don't want you missing yoga!" Dr. G agrees, to my relief.

On the way home, Mitch tells me that his friend Evelyn, a bassoonist who had a mastectomy a few years ago, scolded him when he boasted that he's been coming to the doctors' offices with me. "It's not about *you!*" she chided.

"Evelyn is right," I agree, "though I do appreciate your extraordinary efforts to be at my side." I know how lucky I am to have a husband who's so involved in this process. Bottom line though, cancer is about the cancer patient, and if I were to give in to all the little requests that everyone makes of me ("oh, have another glass of wine," or "this teensy slab of red meat won't hurt you") I'd soon be compromising the things I've decided to do for my health. So if "this is about *me*" means getting to bed early, eating whole, organic foods, taking supplements, walking daily, meditating, practicing yoga, or standing on my head (perhaps *particularly* standing on my head) that's exactly what I'm going to do.

Jill talks about worrying today, and how the asanas help clear the mind. "Eventually that freedom from worry will follow you off your mats, and you'll be able to look at life without constantly being in a state of flight or fright," she explains.

Amen to that!

Of course, I carry her lesson along to radiation later today, a planning session or "simulation," during which the technicians pinpoint the area of the breast to be treated. I figure I'll use my ujjayi breathing, and it will be a piece of cake. I happily kiss Mitch good-bye at the door (spouses are not allowed in the room for this one). I guess that should be a clue, because why *would* they want a spouse in the room when they're planning to subject a patient to torture?

They *do* admit this will be the longest period of holding still during the course of the six-week treatment—twenty minutes, a short break, and then thirty minutes more— but they don't mention that my elbow will be crooked over my head and my fingers and arm will completely fall asleep. They neglect to reveal that I'll feel virtually paralyzed during the process of fitting the "mold" or "immobilization device" to my upper body. (This is supposed to ensure that the patient will be in precisely the same position for every treatment.)

I can't touch my fingers to one another because I can't even move them, and my "Sa, Ta, Na, Ma" self-relaxation method won't work. (I've learned, by the way, that this gibberish actually means something: Sa-Infinity, Ta-Life, Na-Death, Ma-Rebirth; the creation cycle.) This seems worse than labor; at least you can *wiggle* in childbirth. I'm ready to rip this contraption off and make a mad dash for the door.

The two men working on me—one of whom is the spit'n image of a blond Jim Carrey—have some sort of comedy shtick going on. They're wisecracking in a friendly manner, until they realize that *I'm* not kidding, that I'm *really* ready to rip off the damn mold and bolt. Then they get huffy, and threaten, "If you don't behave yourself we'll have to start all over again from the beginning!" By now I'm chanting "Sa, Ta, Na, Ma" so frantically they must think I'm totally berserk. Forget the mold; just bring on a straightjacket!

They have to start over because the first mold isn't fitting right. Neither is the second. Finally, they're satisfied with the third try, and they leave me alone on the table (stepping into one of those little side rooms with the creepy one-way window) while their equipment scans slowly across me, a few feet above my body. I'm not to breathe too deeply ("What's with the *breathing?*" one calls out nastily on the intercom.) So much for ujjayi—I'm not to move even a big toe.

Next, Jim Carrey has the nerve to brand my breast with seven *permanent* tiny blue tattoos. The size of pinheads, they're just to ensure that everything is measured to perfection (and to assure that radiation will never be applied again to this area in the future), but by the time these jokers return me to my husband, I feel like I've been on holiday in Hell.

"Are you all right?" Mitch asks when I emerge from the treatment room, my hair disheveled, and my cheery little gown all crooked and rumpled as if these guys have had their way with me. I slump into my husband's arms.

Later, at home, an employee from the treatment center calls to inform me that my insurance won't cover radiation. "What am I supposed to do now? *Die?*" I demand indignantly.

"Maybe you could qualify as a charity case?"

"I'm a freelance writer, not a bag woman."

Mitch snatches the phone away and the two of them chat calmly. We are covered, after all. Apparently, the insurance companies just get some kind of twisted pleasure from scaring people.

Tomorrow, I'm to show up for a CAT scan. If Carrey steps within a foot of me, I swear it's over. This has been one of the most horrific days I've had in the past two months…but just in a physical sense; my mind feels fairly at ease right now, for some inexplicable reason.

In the morning, I set out again for the radiation center for my CAT scan. This time—not to be fooled (unlike George Bush)—I've taken a Xanax. But like George Bush, I'm fooled again. The technicians are lying in wait for me, though today I don't have to hold the armpit asana for more than a few minutes. I've sedated myself with drugs for no reason.

Before I'm dismissed, a nurse grills me about my various habits, discovering that I'm popping a long list of supplements. "You're taking *what?*" she cries. "No, dear, not with radiation."

Much to my dismay, it turns out most of my supplements are not to be ingested during treatment, for fear that their antioxidant powers will somehow confuse the radiation's attack on the cancer cells. Don't ask me how or why this could possibly happen, but that's the theory (which sounds as reasonable as leech therapy to me). Still, I don't want to rock the tippy cancer boat, so I'll put my peppy little pills aside for the time being.

Today in class, Jill reminds us that we should love ourselves. It's hard to do sometimes, especially when you're overweight or impatient, or when you have a debilitating disease, or even a life-threatening disease. It's hard to say to yourself, "You're lovely, you're perfect" when you know damn well you have millions of flaws. But these flaws aren't really us, Jill claims. At our very center is a perfect, divine being. That's the person we need to honor and love—if we can only find her.

In Jeanine's class tonight, I think I'm close. I always feel so comforted here, listening to her gentle, hypnotic voice. For Jeanine, yoga isn't about the postures; it's about self-awareness, and finding the strength and courage to embrace each day. I'm learning from this gentle teacher that being macho on the mat is not the way to understand yoga, or one's self. Before, I viewed yoga as a way to push myself, a way to improve my body. B.K.S. Iyengar said that the asanas "act as bridges to unite the body with the mind, and the mind with the soul." In this dark, quiet room, I do feel as if I'm coming closer to my soul.

I'm ready for another level in my practice, and Jeanine may help me find it. She sits cross-legged on her mat, a beautiful lilac shawl over her shoulders, her silvery-blonde hair framing her face. Her motherly voice, as musical as a wind chime in a gentle breeze, helps us experience the unconditional love we should have for ourselves.

I wonder why Jill and Jeanine have given a similar message on the same day. Do the yoga teachers have talking points they use, like political pundits or Rush Limbaugh, or is it all part of that magical synchronicity that seems to encircle yoga? I suppose by now, I shouldn't be surprised at all that my yoga teachers are in perfect harmony with what I need to know.

Jeanine says that Mercury is in retrograde, which supposedly causes some kind of confusion in our lives. I guess I do feel a bit confused; getting to know and love this new person I've become is quite a challenge. I'm a person with seven pinpoint blue tattoos on my tit, a two-inch scar, and a calendar filled with doctor and treatment appointments, a person who had cancer, a person who may still have some cancer cells lurking around that need to be zapped for survival. I'm a woman I never imagined being, as if my past and future selves have just been introduced at a dance neither one of us really wants to attend. "Who is that awkward kid in the plaid dress?" my future self asks. Never mind; just dance with her, show her the steps.

But according to my yoga teachers, this is really not who I am anyway: we are not our thoughts, our words, or our worries. My divine and perfect self is and always has been here, like a cookie in a jar, waiting for a little kid to reach her hand in and pluck it out. I can almost see myself standing in front of that cookie jar, gathering my courage. We need so much courage just to love ourselves.

March is taking its time. Mitch and I go out for a walk this morning; on a telephone pole in the middle of town we spy a pigeon hawk. We stand for a while watching him preen and squawk. He's about the size of a regular pigeon, though much slimmer.

As we resume our stroll, I look up at the sky, watching the

hawk soar off. I remember what Jill said the other day: "We are all part of the sky; we are all part of everything." It's funny, because just last week I was gazing out my bedroom window, marveling at all the activity up there. Birds kept jetting across my line of vision, followed by planes and fat cumulus clouds. Most of the time, I'm completely unaware of what's going on right above my head.

Today, the sky, the moon, and the sun all seem to converge in my mind as we walk, and it's not surprising when Mitch suddenly says, "Gee, the sky is full of so much activity today!" I've said it before; marriage is a lot like yoga. When you're married a long time, you just start thinking tandem thoughts, which is why, when I'm craving Chinese food for dinner, I just think really hard about it, and often enough, Mitch will come home from the opera carrying a bag of Chinese take-out with his clarinets.

It's windy today, but nearly sixty degrees, and along with birds, bags and branches are flying through the sky. With every step, I think of how happy I am to see another spring, and of how many, many more I want.

Tonight I fall asleep with the curtains open, under a gleaming crescent moon. This leads me to dream about my father, who consulted the moon almost daily. I never knew a man who so loved the moon, who so loved to talk about "the man in the moon," and "green cheese." When I was a child he would often raise me onto his shoulders and carry me outside onto our wrap-around porch to say goodnight to the moon. I absolutely adored my dad, or Daddy, as I called him into his last years, though he was a strict, proper man— a Republican! But he had a soft side he couldn't always conceal, and he was a devoted husband and father. I remember how Mom used to love pussy willows and how my dad always honored that. When we were riding down a country road, all she had to do was cry out, "Pussy willows!" and my father would swing the Chrysler over to the shoulder and race out into the brush to pluck some branches. He didn't build her the Taj Mahal, but he came to a screeching halt for her. Even as a child, I felt in those sweet little buds, so warm and soft to the touch, the strength of their love.

∞

The wine club meets this evening, our annual St Patrick's Day gathering for corned beef, cabbage, Irish soda bread, and of course, wine. I'm nervous for some reason. Actually, I *know* the reason—it's because I'm not drinking that much, and even though no one is talking about politics, I wonder if in my new, uninebriated state, I'll still enjoy these friends. Mitch is at the opera, so I'm here on my own. Other than the cabbage, there's very little on the menu that fits into my natural, whole foods diet.

I decide to have a little of everything, since I don't really think it was over-indulgence in white flour or corned beef (which I've always consumed just once a year) that gave me cancer. If diet were the only culprit, most of these people would long be dead. But they're a merry group, as always, eating and drinking with abandon. Billy tapes a green plastic Shamrock to his fly, and offers to show me his war scars if I'll show him mine. The room erupts in laughter, the best medicine ever.

I sit for a long time with Annie, just talking quietly. She's been having some problems with her foot, and she's contemplating a surgery. We talk about how you never know what's coming next, how we always worry about the wrong things. "I think these 'bad' things happen to help us put things in perspective, to keep us focused on what really matters," Annie says.

When I rise to leave, there are kisses all around, and Fred— my political nemesis, who considers liberals to be the political equivalent of flesh-eating staphylococcus—blurts out that he loves me. It's not often you can find friends who will tell you they love you right out loud in public, in front of their wives, and in mixed company; right-wing, Limbaugh lovers or not. "I love you, too," I tell Fred, and before I know it I'm in the center of a big 'ol Grand Old Party hug.

∞

Tomorrow is the Ides of March, and they've delayed my radiation start once again, so I'm still waiting, though as my friend from yoga says, I'm not waiting for life to happen any more, I *know* it's happening now. Why should I be in a hurry to spend my midmornings in radiation oncology? On the other hand, if any cancer cells are still skulking around in my breast I'd just as soon be rid of them.

Their excuse is that the machine needs to be "serviced." That's not a very reassuring prospect; and it makes me wonder exactly what might happen if the radiation machine *does* have a flat tire in the middle of a treatment. Maybe I'll hear a sizzle and then one of the techs will blurt out, "Oops!"

I hope not. Perhaps the real reason is that Friday is St. Patrick's Day, and the staff just doesn't feel like staying late to conduct my "dry run." Having a dry run on St. Patty's Day seems pretty darn hilarious, anyway.

∞

As I'm eating my morning oatmeal, I realize I'm thinking about the day the technicians made my mold for radiation, recalling how horrid it was to crook my arm over my head for half an hour. I glance down to see that my oatmeal is almost gone and I haven't even tasted it! So *this* is the way we lose the present moment! I pull my thoughts back to the present. I am *here, now*; I am not in radiation oncology.

Outside, the March wind is blowing the branches of a scotch pine I planted twenty years ago. The tree is immense now, though it was just a sapling when my brother gave it to me. The needles are turning and twirling in the wind, and the branches are furling up and down, but the trunk of the tree is solid and still. The tree is now almost thirty feet tall.

I think of what Jeanine says: "We too can be like the swaying tree, with our roots firm and planted." I hear Jill's voice: "What time is it? Now. What day is it? Today." Thank God I'm learning these lessons. My last few bites of my oatmeal taste divine.

Mitch and I walk this afternoon, and we end up arguing about Sam's future. I admit I haven't been thinking about it lately—not only because of my health crisis, but because I don't really want to face the thought of him going away. The other reason is because we don't have all the facts. Yes, he's been accepted at several colleges, but we still await the more "prestigious" universities. Of course, they don't let the kids know until the eleventh hour.

Mitch demands, "How much money are you willing to go into hock for? He's been offered a free ride at a great school in New Jersey. We could easily spare ourselves the loans."

But I don't want to discuss this now. I want to look at the blue sky, and the towering trees, and feel the wind whipping against my skin. I'm training my mind to think of what's happening now, and I don't want to be careening down a hundred other paths, trying to figure out what I will do "if."

What if. I *hate* those two loathsome words.

Oddly, my husband, who is usually so "Zen," is pressing for an answer. I know he's worried about the money (after all, it's he—not I—who supports our family), but I also feel that he's pushing for the answer *he* wants to hear: "No, we won't borrow a lot of money. Sure, Sam will take a free ride." This would certainly take a lot of pressure off our clarinet player.

But I don't give him that answer today. "When we have the facts, we'll make the decision, and not before. Today, I'm just taking a walk, and looking at the sky."

As we walk home in silence, each of us annoyed with the

other, I'm nevertheless proud of myself. In the past, I would have gladly agreed to dissect all the future possibilities, but not now. If Mitch is going to be that way, next time I'll walk alone.

On this cold, sunny March day our yoga class is full. We begin with a forgiveness meditation; Jill asks us to think of someone who's hurt us in some way, and to try forgiving not the action itself, but the person. I can't think of anyone who's seriously "done me wrong." In fact, the only one that comes to mind is me—so I concentrate on some of the topics that I think of whenever I feel angry at myself…breast cancer comes to mind, of course, because it's quite possible that some of my bad habits have put me in this place. On the other hand, it's likely that I'm completely blameless; I might have drunk some tainted Strontium 90 milk when I was a kid, or had too much Jersey water. There's no point in blaming myself for my own disease, so I try to forgive. "Start from today," Jill says, "and go forward."

Jill asks us to wring ourselves out like sponges. We twist and turn and I can feel the energy of twenty women collectively working our butts off. Maybe this cleansing is part of the forgiveness process—I do feel better afterwards.

At home after class, I fiddle around with some newspaper articles, but my mind wanders. Countdown to radiation: two days to go. Sam comes home from school for lunch and checks the mail. No notices from colleges. Not quite yet. Sigh. More waiting for both of us.

"This is starting to get a little aggravating," Sam admits, "this not knowing what I'm going to be doing in the future."

I nod and smile at my son, quoting my yogini friend, "Don't wait for life to happen. Life is happening now."

Sam briefly considers this deep, cosmic truth before he heads back to school. His enlightened response as he steps out the door: "Yeah, whatever. See ya."

∞

Jill asks us, "Could you still be happy if you lost everything you own?" I guess she's getting at the point that happiness comes from within. I agree with this in theory, and I certainly could get along fine without my car, my jewelry, or maybe even my house. But health is another issue. It's hard to imagine how a person can be happy if they're in chronic pain. Nor could I be happy without my children (though I do enjoy my time of solitude when they're at school!).

Tonight is my practice radiation session, and though I've gone over the details with the kids, they seem surprised when I remind them at dinner that I'll be going out to the hospital later.

"Mom, will this treatment hurt your heart?" Ben asks.

I find this astonishing. I wonder if he's been worrying about this for a while, or whether he's just figured out that if radiation is aimed at a woman's breast it can affect other organs as well. This is a topic I hadn't even thought of myself, until Dr. G mentioned that a small portion of the lung does receive radiation during the process. There is actually a device to protect the heart if the left breast needs to be treated. I give Ben a hug and reassure him, "My heart will be just fine."

But as we drive to the hospital, my heart is racing. I know this is just the "practice run," but it's still unsettling.

Inside the radiation unit, I climb onto the table and snuggle into my mold. This stiff piece of foam and I are going to get pretty chummy but I have a feeling the day will come when I'll be thrilled to see it go. In fact, one of the techs has snidely mentioned that I might get to a point where I'll want to run the thing over with my car. As I crook my arm above my head, I can see that day might arrive quite soon.

Once I'm in place, a lovely German technician warns me that

I'll be motionless for about twenty minutes during the simulation and x-rays. "Do you do yoga?" she asks, taking note of the tiny "Oms" embroidered on my socks.

"Yes!" I answer, hoping to have found a yogini soul mate.

"It's not much of a work-out, is it?" she says.

Sweetheart, I beg to differ; clearly she's never met Jill or Ali. I close my eyes and count the minutes till, like a baked potato, I'm "done."

∞

At last—my first day of real radiation. All my friends are saying how brave I am, but the truth is, there's nothing much to radiation, other than holding still. "Is radiation chemo?" someone asks me. "Does it hurt? Does it make your hair fall out? Does it make you really, really tired?"

The answer is no, to all of the above, at least in my experience. I do feel nervous as I enter the radiation oncology department, but mostly I'm worried about how weird it will be to come here for the next six weeks. And, I'm nervous that it won't work. Radiate away, but just hit the target.

I've decided the male technicians are really nice guys. After all, it must be difficult to be the wardens who make the molds in a radiation unit. It's hard to resist equating the discomfort with the person, but really it's not their fault. I don't even mind baring my chest for these guys— I've come to regard my breast more as a sickly child than as a sexual component of my body.

This morning a tall, black woman with deep-set eyes escorts me to the treatment room, and helps me up onto the table. My mold is already waiting for me and the equipment is ready to roll; I just need to be meticulously positioned, a process that can take quite some time, though the radiation itself is on for only a minute or two. As I slide onto the table, the woman clucks, "I see you're wearing your good-luck socks."

"How did you know?" I ask incredulously.

"Honey, why *else* would you wear them?"

So the bright pink, furry socks that my writers' group gave me don't match my black sweats and shoes and I'm not exactly a fashion statement. Cozy footwear or not, when the technician steps out and I'm stuck in my mold like a fly in a web beneath the towering radiation equipment, I feel a moment of inexplicable terror. How can this be happening?

Before I can work myself into a total panic, the vibrant voices of The Four Tops pour into the room over the intercom. One of the guys is piping in Motown, and "Sugar Pie Honey Bunch" swirls and surrounds me. I nearly laugh out loud; instead of "Sa, Ta, Na, Ma," I'll get through this experience with the help of ShaNaNa. "Reach Out, Reach Out!' is next. It's all I can do to hold my pink socks still!

Today, Jill focuses on Pigeon. I have nothing against the pose, though at the beginning you feel like a sweet little bird with your wings folded over your head, and by the end you can hardly flutter.

She attributes her preoccupation with the pose to a book I loaned her last week—Anne Lamott's *Bird by Bird*. One of my favorites, it's about writing, but it's also about any creative pursuit in life. I'm glad that Jill is enjoying it, although the other class members moan and beg me not to give our teacher any more books to read.

On my way out, I decide to apply the concept to my radiation treatments. In her book, Lamott writes about how her brother was overwhelmed by a report he had to complete on all the birds of North America. His dad advised him just to tackle the project "bird by bird." I won't think of thirty-three treatments, I'll just think of one at a time, bird by bird, pigeon by pigeon, rad by rad.

As I enter our house, I nearly trip over a big fat letter addressed to Sam from CMU that's fallen through our mail slot and onto the floor. Big and fat means good news— those slim, flat letters are the ones you have to watch out for. My heart is wild with happiness: he's in! All those years of hard work have paid off. We still haven't heard from Princeton, but Carnegie Mellon is right up there. The waiting, for both of us, is almost over. I'm in the middle of my journey, and he's about to embark on his. Life is happening *now*. I place the envelope on his computer keyboard so he'll see it first thing when he comes home from school.

At Jeanine's class tonight we gather in a circle for a family Tree pose. We wrap our arms around one another, intertwined and strong. Before Savasana, Jeanine distributes mala beads; as we meditate, we pass the beads through our fingers, a soothing sensation. Jeanine suggests we repeat a phrase of our choice as we touch each bead, with every inhale and exhale. I choose "healing strength." I like the two words side by side.

After class, Anneke stops in. "Can we *not* discuss the C word tonight?" I ask before she brings it up.

"Sure, whatever you say," she smiles. It's a relief to sit with my friend and bask in her humor and energy again. I understand what Eloise's sister's friend meant about not talking about the "disease" at every opportunity. It's not that I'm in denial—yes, I'm well aware that I may still have cancer cells in my body, and that's why I'm going to radiation. But I don't want to think about it all the time. I want to sit with one of my very best friends and laugh at her jokes and believe that we'll be together for a long, long time.

Waiting at the hospital for my radiation treatment this morning, I pick up a Glamour magazine that's on a nearby chair. One of the cover blurbs pops out at me: "This is the Year You'll Get a Great Body. And It Will Only Take You Fifteen Minutes a

Day!" I doubt if the editors were referring to radiation treatments when they wrote this blurb, but that's the way I take it. Perhaps a whimsical angel has arranged for me to find it.

My writers' group meets this afternoon. Kayla is beginning a project on women's networking. Jessica is writing about meditation, Amy is working on poetry, and I, of course, am writing about yoga. We're all rejuvenated, as if our invisible muses have awakened from a long winter, brushed themselves off, and taken their places around our table. As we trade stories and laugh, I think about how much these women—my writing sisters— mean to me. I flash back to a meeting we had a year or so ago, when none of us had been writing, and we were considering ending the group. I cried, "We can't do that! I love you all too much!" and within seconds, they all agreed. I'm so glad we've stuck together, even though we're years and, financially at least, worlds apart. (My entire first floor would fit in Jessica's living room, and I could eat off the tiles of her finished basement with its home theatre, bar and sparkling laundry area, whereas even the spiders seem traumatized by the living conditions in *my* cellar.)

Out of curiosity I decide to try Jeanine's regular class tonight. As I sit in cross-legged position the room fills around me, and soon there's hardly space for even one more student. Men and women of all ages come to this class, and they aren't dressed to the yogi nines here. There are women in ragged tees and sweats who look like they've just come from making their family's dinner, and the men are in their fifties, with graying beards. I like this place.

Jeanine leads us through a vigorous vinyasa (flow), swiftly transitioning between poses. This is a very different class than her "stress and healing" session, and some of the movements are difficult, but I do as much as I can. I'm focused on my own mat, honoring my own body. This is definitely not a class for beginners. But—news flash— I am no longer a beginner!

∞

It's the last day of March, and the dreaded slim letter arrives today. Sam is rejected from Princeton. Somehow, the boy takes it well. "Damn," he says, "I don't like rejection."

Well, neither do I.

Neither does anyone, but it's part of life. And after all I've learned this year, I don't think it really matters. I'm just grateful that Gino got accepted at Rutgers and will be able to go. And if I'm doomed to four years of driving Sam to Western Pennsylvania where the signs on the highways actually warn "Beware of Aggressive Drivers" (maybe because there's nothing else to do but go out and drive like a demon in Western Pennsylvania) so be it.

Anyway, as my darling Anneke astutely observes when I tell her the news, "A lot of brilliant people…didn't go to Princeton."

CHAPTER TWENTY-THREE: APRIL

The Remover of Obstacles

Sam will be attending CarNegie Mellon, the school that resembles a blueberry tart. He seems depressed for a day, but it doesn't take long for him to recover. When I email my cousin to tell her the college outcome, she says not to worry; she believes there must be someone very important at CMU that Sam is meant to meet, because everything happens "for a reason." A year or so ago, I would have laughed that email right out of my inbox, but now I have to agree.

After my treatment today, Mitch and I meet up for lunch with his carpool musicians—a French horn player, a violist, and the bassoonist, Evelyn, who has had a mastectomy and is coming up on her second year of being cancer free. The four all play at the opera and ballet; they drive into the City together to save on tolls and parking fees.

Evelyn leans toward me, across the table. "I joined a group online of a dozen breast cancer survivors. They're from all over the country, but we recently got together in Chicago! It was wonderful; we wore pink hats to identify each other at the airport!"

"Wow, that's great! I haven't really felt the urge to join any support groups," I confess, "but I have my writers' group and book club, and my wine club, too. They all keep me laughing and busy."

Evelyn nods approvingly, "Whatever works for you!" She explains that the women in her group all happen to have a particular type of breast cancer that's not estrogen receptor positive, and can't be treated with a hormone therapy pill. Evelyn had a lumpectomy, then a recurrence in the other breast, a mastectomy and reconstructive surgery. She's newly a grandmother, with soft brown eyes and strong opinions.

For the first time in nearly thirty years of dining with musicians, the conversation doesn't even touch upon conductors or performances. It's all about Evelyn and me, and how we've coped with the disease of breast cancer. I can't believe that I'm sitting at a table of musicians and we're not even talking about reeds or tone. Rather, the other carpool members seem totally mesmerized by our conversation; I think they've been wanting Evelyn to open up to them more, and having me here is allowing this to happen.

As we walk back to our cars, Evelyn places her arm around my shoulder, "One day, you'll see; you'll wake up and the first thing you think about will *not* be breast cancer."

Funny. I was just wondering this morning when that might happen. Not for a long time, I'd wager, but it's good to hear from a "true expert" that the day will come.

∞

It's the first Sunday of the month, and tonight is the meditation circle; I give it a second try, even though Jeanine isn't leading. We have another facilitator tonight, a young woman who seems to know all the ins and outs of the world of yoga; she distributes copies of words to chant in "Pali," said to be the language of the Buddha, more ancient than Sanskrit. One of the meditations for tonight is a "loving-kindness" meditation, called "metta" in Pali, in which we're to silently repeat loving wishes for ourselves, then for the world, and then for someone we don't like. This is perfect, since Friday at school Sam got into some trouble because he "made a face" at one of our administrators. I close my eyes, envisioning the assistant principal, wishing her a peaceful heart, a healthy body, and a life of loving kindness, wishing that in her peaceful state she'll decide not to call Sam into her office on Monday as she's threatened, not to yell at him for caring enough about a perceived injustice involving some members of his baseball team to have an "unhappy look" on his face. I've been thinking of marching into her office first thing tomorrow and giving her a piece of my mind, anyway. It hadn't occurred to me that a piece of my mind might literally be incarnated in a "loving kindness" meditation, and this brings a smile to my lips. We'll see if it works.

Jill is back from another yoga journey to California, where she's learned to surf. She says she felt incredibly powerful on the surfboard, and encourages us to use positive words when we think of ourselves. "I am what?" she asks, " I am powerful, strong, healthy, beautiful!"

So often we use negatives to describe ourselves. I think of the words I've been using lately: *I am safe; I am strong.* I hope that words can change or create reality. I'd like to believe that *thoughts* could change reality.

Jill says that her roommate on the outing wanted to gain wisdom, and at the end of the week, another yogini commented to Jill, "Your roommate is so wise!" Jill believes that we really create our own realities. I wonder if this can be true of our health.

At radiation today, I feel myself tensing as the technician positions my body and explains that he'll be taking x-rays of my breast before proceeding with the treatments. So once again, I'm not to move at all for at least twenty minutes with my elbow crooked over my head in the damn mold. Holding still is my greatest physical challenge right now. I just keep hearing Jill's sweet voice: "Go to the breath."

I look deeply into this technician's eyes and think about what boyish, long lashes he has, and I try to remember that he's not a prison warden but a young man who's here to help me on this journey. Without a word, he gently adjusts my robe, and my mind calms: I am motionless on the table, my breathing steady. If my mother could see me now, she'd be weeping with fear. "It's okay, Mom," I'm thinking. "Honest."

Back home, I ask Sam how things worked out with the assistant principal. She hasn't called him into her office; apparently, she's decided to let the whole thing slide!

∞

I'm feeding Beth's cat for her this week, since she's gone on vacation. The cat no longer frightens me, nor do I fear getting murdered while I'm in Beth's empty apartment. I'd like to dare a burglar to come after me while I'm feeding Arlo. I'm so bold these days that if anyone crosses me here I'll just pick up the disgusting kitty litter tray and use it as a lethal weapon!

Arlo rubs against me as I bend to fill his dish; he doesn't swat at my legs or try to bite me as he used to. He must sense that I'm someone he can't mess with anymore. Even the cat sees me as a changed woman.

"Bye, sweet little kitty," I joke as I lock Beth's door behind me.

I make it to Jill's class on time; her theme today is "honor the teacher within." We all have a lot to teach ourselves, but like kids in a classroom we're often throwing spitballs or daydreaming. It's hard to pay attention to our inner voice.

During our poses, Jill instructs me several times to keep my belly in. Since I hardly even have a belly any more—giving up my wine and the stress of cancer have resulted in the loss of that menacing final five pounds of unwanted weight—I find this comical. I tuck in my tush *and* my belly, happily adjusting my Warrior. In a class of twenty, I no longer even care if my belly is mentioned.

After class, Jill calls me over. "You've inspired me to sign up for a creative writing class!" she whispers shyly.

"Fantastic! Is this because you read *Bird by Bird*?"

"I think so!"

It's somehow touching that she's going to follow in my footsteps for a bit; I've been following in hers for nearly two years now. I'm glad I gave her that book to read.

Tonight, Jeanine places a rhythmic CD on the CD player and leads us in a class that seems more like creative dance than yoga. "You won't find these poses in the yoga handbook," Jeanine admits, telling us to bend and sway the way the music moves us, to snake our hands in our Warrior poses, to circle our hips and follow our own impulses. I close my eyes and melt into the movements, so grateful to be here. I *do* honor the teacher within, but I'm also acutely aware of how blessed I am to have Jeanine and Jill in my life.

On the way out, I chat with Jeanine a bit and learn that she's about as fond of George Bush as I am. We imagine what a yoga class with Bush and Cheney would be like, and we're laughing in each other's embrace as we construct a dialogue in which our President and Vice President maneuver into Downward Dog: "Heh, heh, Dick, does that Dog go up or down?" It's a funny sight to imagine. But in all seriousness, we agree that if politicians were required to practice yoga, the world would be a very different place. The credo of the true yogi, after all, is ahimsa: to do no harm.

∞

At the Jazz Band dinner—an annual early April event in support of our young high school musicians, Sam on his trumpet among them—my friend Anise from the wine club is having a meltdown because her son wants to attend another high school next year. The club always reserves a table for this BYOB event, held in a dingy church basement.

"I'll miss all my friends," she complains. "And I won't get to help on the fundraisers like this one. I won't know *anyone* at that other school!"

"There's a reason why he wants to switch to the 'tech' school. Maybe it's just meant to be. And you can still keep in touch with everyone—we'll certainly still be friends," I reassure her.

"I know," she says sadly.

"Besides," I joke, "You can always come back and help with our fundraisers!" We spent hours this afternoon hanging balloons and pasting fake palm trees on the walls.

"*Right,*" Anise frowns.

"I just *know* it's going to be fine."

"I'm not so sure. And anyway, it just won't be the same. Look at those seniors up on the stage! Soon they'll all be gone. Why does everything have to change?" Anise asks tearfully.

When I gaze up at Sam and Gretchen on the stage, blasting their trumpets side by side, I know that if I go down the road that Anise is on, my heart will burst with pain. I don't believe that our hearts are *meant* to burst with pain, but if we can't learn this lesson—the lesson of change—sorrow is the outcome. I'm convinced that's what happened when my mother died: even though she was eighty-one and had lived a long, happy life filled with family and love, I wasn't ready to let her go, and so my heart and body did literally explode with pain, and eventually with disease. Maybe that's crazy, but it's what I now believe.

After all, even a surgeon can't know when cancer really appeared. I suspect my tumor began the day my mother died or that the malignant cells began to merrily convene in the months that followed, when my thoughts were so painful and hopeless. Or maybe the cells began on our Vermont vacation, the week before her death, on the day Mom collapsed while I was washing her hair at the kitchen sink. I called out to Mitch for help, and as "luck" would have it he raced outside to find that the woman in the very next cabin was a nurse and a man just around the bend was an EMT. Within moments, they were at my side, able to take over and revive my mother even before an ambulance arrived.

My mother needed to say good-bye to her family; and so in the week that followed, my sister flew east from Arizona, where she was then living, and my brother came from upstate New York; my niece returned and my nephews came from far and wide. They all headed to Burlington, to be at the hospital as my mother's mystery illness unraveled. Maybe this is when my cancer began; it's certainly when my general outlook—always hovering on the brink of fear and disaster—turned to a dramatic downward spiral.

But now my spiral is headed upwards. Sam—in his Hawaiian shirt and sunglasses, in keeping with the evening's decorating theme—belts out a gorgeous solo and even in this room full of parents and kids he finds me with his gaze and flashes me an intoxicating smile. Should I let that smile break my heart, or should I let it give me all the strength that a child's love can offer? Well, okay, a little of both, but I'm going to be strong in my emotions, as well as in my body, and I'm going to believe that though we can't hold forever onto the moment, we can choose to be completely in it, and to honor it with our full attention and respect.

Eva, who's sitting across from me, announces that she's painted me a picture (she studied art in college, though she hasn't pursued her interest professionally). I'm so touched that I vow to myself that no matter what it looks like—and I've never seen Eva's work before—the painting is going up in my living room. I'm just grateful to learn it's a snowscape and not a portrait of her beloved President.

∞

Ben is fifteen today. There's no school this week, so I let him sleep in while I head to yoga. I remember the day he was born, after a warm, flowery morning and an afternoon thunderstorm. The weather that day seemed like pre-arranged fanfare for his birth, with the warm, gentle breeze blowing, and then a magnificent storm. I recall coming home and placing him in the arms of Aaron and Sam who were seated on the couch, seven and three, respectively; a new brother to share, and that's just what they did.

I'm early for yoga today, and Jill greets me with tales from her writing class (apparently, the participants are septuagenarians, writing their memoirs for their grandchildren!) She also hands me a package.

"What's this?" I ask.

"Just a little gift. You'll see."

I open the box and pull out a small statue. I'm delighted, and confused. "Who—or what— is it?"

"He's my favorite," Jill explains. "The Hindu deity, Ganesh. He's known as the Remover of Obstacles. The son of Lord Shiva and the goddess Parvati—I've heard a number of stories about his birth—he has an elephant head and though he's rather obese, he balances on a mouse. See? In his right hand he holds a goad, which is supposed to propel us on the eternal path while removing obstacles. In his left hand he grasps a noose—this supposedly captures the difficulties. He should be placed facing the front door."

"The remover of obstacles! I like that. Thank you!" I smile and hug Jill. I'm more excited to have a Ganesh statue than a priceless jewel. I feel as if she's letting me know that *she* knows I get it. I'm a true believer in the power and purpose of the universe now—no more iceberg theories for me.

With Jill's help, I hold a Handstand today for all of ten seconds! Even with my newfound slim and shapely body, resting my weight on my hands and arms feels a lot like lifting a refrigerator packed full of meat and ice. It's amazing that I can walk around all day carrying this weight without any problem.

When I get home, I search for an appropriate place for Ganesh, who's incredibly heavy considering the fact that he's only about seven inches tall. I had thought of hanging him on a wall, but were he to fall, that might be the end of someone I love. This is the same reason I put my Buddha in a glass case—he (or she) is about two feet high and really could do some damage.

I hold the elephant-god in my hands and survey the room. I try the coffee table, but that seems a little ostentatious. I turn, and my gaze rests on the obvious choice—a marble table my mother bequeathed to me—which is now full of pictures of the kids. But it also holds two wonderful little carved elephants Ruthann brought me from a trip to India. Ganesh looks quite comfortable between them, and he's also perfectly positioned to face the entryway. Yes, I realize that obstacles make life interesting, but it's their removal, in some cases, that enables life to go on.

In the afternoon, Ben and I head out to a nearby restaurant for a birthday lunch. As we walk to our destination a light rain picks up and I pull out my umbrella. Ben takes the umbrella and holds it in his hand above our heads, protectively placing his arm around my waist as we snuggle together to stay dry. I'm in awe of this moment, and filled with love for my growing son, who isn't too cool to put his arm around his mom and hold her close.

∞

The moon is full tonight and surrounded by a ring of blue haze. My bedroom windows are open, and I can hear voices from the house next door; the former owners have moved away (failing to make a Zen garden, or any kind of garden), and a new family with a slew of teenagers has moved in. The magnolia tree is in full bloom, and the pear blossoms are white. The apple tree—which cracked during a winter storm—is blossoming, too, after we plied it with tree medicine and roped its falling branches together, hoping for its revival. I hear Sam's trumpet blasting into the night; he and Gretchen broke up a few days ago. This is disappointing for him, but it also means he's home more.

As of today, I'm halfway through my radiation treatments. In some ways, it feels as if I'm perpetually in that nightmare mold; my breast has turned a bright, rashy red, as if I've been sunbathing topless (not very likely, especially now that my right breast resembles a defective pancake). In other ways, it's just a minor inconvenience; for an hour a day I'm occupied with getting to and from the hospital. A lovely young radiology therapist named Denise, who's pregnant with her third child, has been assigned to watch over me. She calls me "gorgeous" and "honey" and treats me like a queen. I've purchased half a dozen fuzzy socks for good luck, and when I climb up onto the table and place my arm overhead, my socks always inspire admiration— even from the male attendants.

I've read that women feel cut adrift when their treatments end, their doctor visits taper off, and they're left to wonder if and when their cancer will return. I can see why.

It's easy to sit here pondering that unanswerable question; or, I can sit here and listen to a distant train, trumpet blasts, Ben whistling as he plays on his computer, and Aaron's footsteps as he gets ready for bed. I'd rather think of the man in the moon than cancer cells. Directing my thoughts is an art I have yet to master, but I'm learning.

In *What We Ache For*, a book I'm reading before turning out my light, I've come across an exercise: Imagine you could erase one year of your life, and how that might change everything that comes later.

One would think *this* would be the year that I'd erase, and yet I have learned so much. I would rather erase the year of my mother's death.

A family first. Mitch is working and the kids decide we'll go out; Aaron is paying with his credit card since he's recently gotten a raise. As the waiter seats us, I can't believe that I'm old enough to have three young men—my sons—accompany me to dinner, and pick up the tab.

Naturally, one thought leads to another and before I know it, I'm thinking about Sam going off to Pittsburgh in a few months, and how empty the house will feel without him—just as it did when Aaron left—and soon there are tears in my eyes and I'm neglecting to pay attention to the glorious experience of dining out with my three sons, who are no longer spilling their milk, throwing food, or kicking each other under the table.

When the boys were young, I had a recurring vision, like a dream of a place you've never been but know you'll one day see. It was of the five of us sitting at a table, the kids with size thirteen feet; long, hairy legs that hung over the chairs, gruff voices, hard, calloused hands. As my sons coarsened, Mitch and

I softened, our skin creased and pallid, our hair fringed with gray. In the vision, our kids weren't throwing their food on the floor; they were drinking milk from oversized jugs, asking for steak, demanding that I order two or three pizzas with all the trimmings. They weren't pulling each other's hair or spitting Cheerios at the window; they were arguing about Dante and swapping bets on the Knicks. Mitch and I gazed at each other across our table, now grown too small for our cumbersome family—and I was in tears. Where have my little boys gone, I wondered; what has become of me?

This is the vision that wrenched my heart—simply the vision of our future. It's the one that cropped up when the boys were screaming and fighting over the last orange Popsicle, when they wrecked their new toys or wiped wet, green toothpaste on the bedroom wallpaper. Just when I wanted to wave a wand and make them disappear, I would see this scene and realize that I didn't have to wave a wand after all; they were already going.

I imagine my mom turned her vision of *my* childhood over and over like a precious stone in the hazed light of memory to see it glisten, for my mother didn't like change any more than I, and she tried to hold onto everything in her life—her husband, her children, her home, her youth—for as long as she possibly could. My mother was girlish well into her seventies; when she answered the phone you might have guessed you were hearing the sweet, lilting tone of a child. She spoke as she swam—which is the way I swim also since she taught me how—in smooth sidestrokes, stopping now and then to float on her back, looking up into the clouds passing over the sunlight. My mother and I never put our faces in the water, never glided forcefully with our arms stretching out ahead. We didn't jump off diving boards, or kick our feet. Just the sidestroke, bit by bit, then we'd stop to float. That's how we swam; that's how we made things last.

Sam senses that my thoughts are headed in a melancholy

direction and draws me back. "I'm scared Carnegie Mellon will be too hard," he confesses. "The architecture majors said sometimes they cry themselves to sleep at night."

"You can handle it," I reassure him. "What was it Dad and I advised *you*, Aaron, when you went off? There are three essential things to remember about college. Just make sure you get enough rest, enough food, and…and…what was the third one?"

I'm stymied for a moment, and Aaron seems to be, too. Was it exercise?

"Use condoms?" Ben asks.

"Yeah, that's it," I nod. "And always use condoms."

Thanks to the thought of my sons having sex, I'm totally *here* now. No more worrying about the future or past.

∞

In mid-April the trees are bright green with the first spring leaves; yoga is fun today, and I feel up to the challenges. Jill is building our arm and core strength, and she alternates between an elbow-supported one legged Plank and a Downward Dog, asking us to hold each pose for five breaths, then going back and forth between the two.

Of course, Jill gives us a spiritual pep talk before class, reminding us that we need to face the hard things in life, and not run away from them. The difficult experiences allow us to really appreciate the easier times, she notes, and then, as if to illustrate, she leads us through the Plank/Dog sequence. By the time we get to a Child's Pose, we are indeed grateful to be there.

She also talks about the Three Poisons— desire, hatred and ignorance. Buddhists say we must be aware of these in order to reach a higher spiritual state. I can't really relate to some of this, but I do know what my teacher means when she says we should try to be less attached to outcomes, objects, and even to others. I certainly have an attachment problem when it comes to my kids—separation anxiety isn't just for five-month-old babies; it's also for aging moms.

I'm not thinking yogic thoughts later today when the therapists have difficulty positioning me for radiation. Out of the blue, my ten-minute session turns into an hour, and I revisit the same discomfort and panic I felt on that first mold-making day. Things we take for granted, like being able to put your damn arm wherever you please, gain a whole new importance when they're denied.

Billy stops by tonight for coffee, and I don't want to complain about my day since he seems so visibly relieved when he sees me. "You look great!" he cries, pointing out that I'm getting a tiny bit of belly back. "You were wasting away there, for a while. You had me worried." Billy is a tall man with a lean, sturdy frame, but he likes women with a little "meat on their bones."

Mitch sits with us, sipping coffee and eating cake that Billy has brought. Billy says his business—which has something to do with computers—"sucks" these days, but of course he's not blaming Bush for the economy. I'll never turn Billy into a liberal, and he'll never turn me into a Republican; that's just the way it's going to be. It's a miracle that we're on the same page about anything. But maybe it's that quality of loyalty to GW that also makes him such a steadfast friend to me.

After Billy leaves, I step out onto our deck. I notice that there are more blossoms on the apple tree this year than ever, as if its brush with death after that winter storm has made it want to flower even more profusely. If it's possible to know just how a tree feels, then I think I do.

∞

I sit with Sam at his computer today, taking a "virtual tour" of the dorms at CMU, trying to pick out a room for the fall. I find it amazing that kids can actually peek inside the dorms on their home computers, panning the rooms, checking out the fitness centers and pool tables. We've been working toward this since his first day of preschool, and here it is.

After we pick out a dorm, I drive to the grocery store in the rain. A Crosby, Stills and Nash song comes on the radio, and as I loop the streets in my van, the beauty of the rain-soaked flowering trees overcomes me. The blossoms are heavy, drooping, laden with color. Purple, pink, orange, violet, white; at every house there's another tree, another shade, another variety of flowering tree. I pull up to a stop sign; there's no car behind me, so I just sit, gazing at a pink dogwood that's spread like a fan in front of a small, Victorian-era house. So many times I've driven by this spot on my way to the grocery store without pausing.

Our wine club meets tonight. We gather around Robin's baby grand piano with our glasses and appetizers listening to Billy Joel on the CD player, a singer I must admit I totally missed during the height of his popularity in the Eighties. I was raising Aaron then; changing diapers, breastfeeding, trying to write magazine columns with a toddler around my ankles. Listening to Billy Joel or anyone else was not on my agenda.

I look around the room at this ragtag group. Mitch is moping in a corner, uncomfortable with the conversations about immigration and taxes. But then politics are cast aside, and Annie pretends to play along with "Piano Man," and we all sing or hum along with the music, and I realize that this crazy group that I've been getting together with now for seven years, is really not so unlike a family, really not so unlike my *own* family.

Maybe this is part of the reason I tend to gravitate toward right-wingers; it's a perfect re-creation of the political climate of my childhood. At our family gatherings, liberals and conservatives were always sparing as they shared the holiday turkey. Even my parents—as much as she adored my father, my mother always voted Democrat—were polar opposites, politically. Dad was a

Nixon man.

Tonight, when I crawl into bed, I listen to the rain pulsing against the window, and in the dim light, I open an Anne Tyler novel. It's been a long time since I've wanted to read fiction. I remember that my mother stopped reading before she died. She even refused when I asked if she wanted me to read aloud to her in the hospital; I had purchased the fifth book in the Jan Karon series she loved, hoping to trick her back into life with tales of Father Tim, the Episcopalian rector, and she wasn't buying. Without words, she was giving me the message she didn't have enough time left for reading.

I feel so comforted in bed tonight with my book.

We concentrate on our hands today in yoga, and Jill has us attempting Crow on two blocks, paying attention to how our weight is distributed as we press firmly. In Savasana, Jill tells us to place our right hand over our heart, and then rest our left hand on top of it; then she begins the three reps of "Om." From this position, I can feel my body vibrating with sound, and the Oms coming from around me seem louder than usual. I love the feeling of connection between the earth, my heart, and the other voices. It's a powerful way to end our practice.

When I get home, Mitch is standing forlornly in the doorway. "Aunt Hannah died," he says as I come in. I put my arms around him and we hug for a moment; in his embrace, I find myself wishing that his beloved aunt, his mother's sister, will find her parents, her husband, and all the souls she has loved in the past. I honestly don't buy into the Heaven concept, or most of what I've ever learned at church, but my newfound connection with the universe is giving me permission to imagine that there's something that exists beyond our earthly understanding.

I guess by rejecting organized religion and all its rules and fairytales, I was also limiting my own capacity to hope. There can't be anything "after," I would tell myself. It isn't logical. Now that I've awakened my spiritual side, I'm open to possibility. As Jill says, to believe that there is something, "All you have to do is look at the sky."

I like what one of Mitch's musician friends, a soulful trumpet player, says about the various religions: "I believe *everything*. I believe in it *all*."

∞

The month is nearly over, and I have only eight more radiation treatments to go! Mitch has come with me whenever he can, sitting in the waiting room, sipping coffee while I disappear into "the room." This is yet another advantage of being married to a musician, even though I'm perfectly capable of going on my own. The staff seems impressed that I arrive most days with my loyal bodyguard.

Today, jubilant that the end is near, I'm fixated on the word "bosom." As we drive home from the hospital I consider the word, contemplating why it's gone out of fashion. Whatever happened to bosom, the word that so fascinated me when I was a child? I remember a little friend once commenting that my mother had "big bosoms," an observation that sent my modest mom scurrying from the room in shock and embarrassment. I remember, too, the day my father read the opening paragraph of *The Legend of Sleepy Hollow* to me aloud. "In the bosom of one of those spacious coves which indent the eastern shore of the Hudson…" uttered aloud by my proper, straight-laced father nearly caused me to dive, blushing, beneath the kitchen table. He pronounced the word "boo-zum," which I found all the more horrifying. Beth and I loved to privately call one another "bosom buddies" when we were youngsters, erupting into girlish, uncontrollable giggles at the very sound of the word. But alas, bosom seems to have retired. Replaced, everywhere I go, by breast. Breast reduction, breastfeeding, breast implants, breast enhancement. Breast… cancer.

I suppose it doesn't matter, and as I rant on and on about this, Mitch just shakes his head.

Later, I opt for Jeanine's more vigorous class, placing my mat next to a bearded, middle-aged man and settling in. Tonight, she focuses on the Backbend, which is not my favorite asana. Even worse, to my horror, she suggests we try a partner pose.

"One partner," Jeanine explains, "will fold into Child's pose while the other bends backwards over her, stretching arms overhead so that the other partner can grab her hands and pull her even more deeply into the stretch."

Just one problem: my partner is a *guy*. The nearest women have already teamed up, leaving me with this gray-haired fellow. He looks at me expectantly, and asks, "Would you like to go first?"

Miraculously, I'm not too self-conscious to comply. "Sure!" I say, and as he bends into Child's pose beneath me, I stretch my body above him, neatly fitting along the length of his spine. Believe it or not, this pose feels great.

Then we switch places, and I'm "on the bottom." My partner is a small man, but with a yogi's muscles, and I can feel his weight as he bends across me (a non-yogi just might think we are testing out a page from *The Joy of Sex*), but I can withstand it, and soon enough we're back in our proper places. I'll definitely have to try this at home with Mitch.

I've successfully negotiated an intimate yoga pose with a stranger, but I can't help wondering how I'll feel if I ever run into this dude in the grocery store. Will I skulk away, or yell out, "Hey, remember me? I'm the babe who jumped on your bones at yoga!"

∞

My last session with the evil mold! Denise, my radiation therapist, smiles as she positions me. The last few treatments, called "the boost," will be done without my chummy contraption. "From now on you'll just have to recline on your side like Cleopatra! It will be a snap!"

This seems almost too good to be true. No more mold; no more arm above the head? I'm afraid to trust that it could be "easy" from now on. Maybe she forgot to mention that they'll be sticking pins in my feet while I'm in Cleopatra pose, or I'll be on my side but submerged under water holding my breath like David Blaine.

"The worst is over," Mitch reassures me as I come out from my treatment, tucking a stray wisp of hair behind my ear. I do so hope he's right.

Tonight we attend the opening of an art exhibit focused on breast cancer in a nearby town. A local sculptress has made, ironically enough, "molds" from breast cancer survivors. I'm going to make a mold myself, a fact which thoroughly grosses out my children when they ask what that plaster kit is doing on the dining room table. But I have to wait until radiation is over; right now my breast is radish red and sensitive to touch.

The artist is an elegant woman dressed in black and strapped heels. High school girls wearing pink tees recite the testimonials of the women who have offered their breasts up to art, women of all ages, with various experiences, but all who seem to have the same message: breast cancer is hardly a gift, but it does make one resoundingly appreciate the precious nature of life. As the girls take turns rising to read their scripts, I notice many of the women in the audience are in tears. It's both upsetting and comforting to hear how others unknown to you have shared your fear and pain. A woman in deep purple with a head of curly blonde hair is weeping, holding her husband's arm tightly. I grasp Mitch's hand.

Yes, we've all been through a lot, and seeing these mounted plaster breasts, hearing the words of women who have gone through surgery, chemo, and radiation, who have wondered if they'll be alive to see their child's next birthday or to hold their grandchildren, is heartbreaking.

The show is sad but oddly fascinating. Mitch and I scrutinize the breast plasters, commenting on how the surgeries have affected the shape and contour, as if we're at the Metropolitan Museum of Art, scratching our heads and remarking upon Van Gogh's dynamic use of color. Some are completely flattened; others look almost "normal." Each breast is slightly different, as is each woman's experience with breast cancer. All that we share is the fear, uncertainty, and a necessary courage.

We introduce ourselves to the artist, then stroll outside to a gazebo to watch as the sun sets, marveling as the light flickers over the leaves of a giant copper beech. Just as the sun dips out of sight, we start home.

Before bed, I decide I'll rise early in the morning to have some quiet time and get a good start on the day. I pick up the Jack Kornfield book I'm reading, and as "coincidence" would have it, open to a selection about getting up early to meditate and start the day mindfully! Why am I not surprised?

CHAPTER TWENTY-FOUR: MAY

Breath of Joy

We're walking today and Mitch breaks into a skip. He's been doing this frequently of late, just to get me laughing. There's nothing funnier than seeing a grown man with a long gray ponytail skipping down the sidewalk swinging his arms. Especially someone like my husband, who is normally anything but "loose" with his movements. Invariably, I collapse into laughter when he does this, begging him to stop as if I'm a mortified adolescent.

I ask Mitch if he did a lot of skipping in his childhood, if he was a happy child. I know he was, but somehow I don't think he had quite the babying that I did; he was allowed to roam more, and his sisters got the lion's share of his parents' attention. In my home, my brother and sister were so much older that I often felt like an only child; I had the best of both worlds, really, because my siblings came in handy when I needed them, but when I was little my parents were very focused on me. Always, I felt warm and protected; my mother was forever at home and my father worked nine to five. I loved my childhood so much I never wanted to grow up. I spent hours at the stained glass window on the stairwell; when I looked through the red pane the yard took on a religious glow as if Christ had been crucified in the fiery rose bed, the crimson blades of grass burning up to his ankles. If I looked through the blue pane, the yard was majestic and serene—still, like a swimming pool at night, lit only by fireflies, or lightning bugs as my father always called them. I spent whole mornings in my imaginary backyard house under the dogwood trees, hours on my seesaw and swing with my father, or drawing and playing paper dolls with my mother who never uttered a harsh or critical word. I was treated like a beloved princess.

I hear often of people who had horrible childhoods, but mine was idyllic, filled with love and care. Mitch says that's all very nice, but maybe my parents didn't really prepare me for adulthood. They certainly didn't prepare me for independence, or taking risks. Yet they gave me two essential ingredients: love and the time to be a child.

Today is the first "boost"—a quick treatment in the radiation room— in "Cleopatra position," just as Denise promised. A friendly technician dots my boob with a blue pen, positions me on my side, and slips out for a few moments. The radiation machine zaps on, and I freeze, listening to piped in Sinatra. On the ceiling there's a woodland scene someone has painted to distract the patients. I concentrate, of course, on the butterfly, and before I know it, I'm done.

We drive back home, but before I enter the house I quickly slip into the backyard to check on my patient. Low and behold, the apple tree is still hanging on to its flowering petals, sweeping its branches toward the earth like a ballet dancer taking an elegant bow.

∞

I'm not surprised that Jill focuses on childhood at our class today! I'm so used to this sort of thing happening that I almost expect it now. If you look for patterns and connections you will find them; if you choose not to see, then that's exactly it, you're choosing. In the past I would deny these things because they didn't seem logical or possible. Now I simply accept.

Jill says that when we're small children, we're curious and trusting, open to new experiences. "We can be children on our mats," she says as we pull our legs into Happy Baby pose. "We can know the freedom of a child, without worrying about what someone else is thinking."

I close my eyes and imagine Mitch skipping down the street. But I wonder, once you've faced cancer, if you can ever truly be child-like again.

I have two yoga classes today: Jill's and Jeanine's, but I don't seem to feel particularly rejuvenated after either one. Now, I'm worrying about the *end* of radiation. I have only two sessions left, and then I'll be cut loose. Dr. G says she'll meet with me one more time for a follow up, and then she hopes to never see me again. As much as I like her, the feeling is mutual.

Tonight, Jeanine instructs, "Breathe in a word that you want to be and breathe out a quality you want to get rid of."

I try various combinations: breathe in courage, breathe out fear; breathe in strength, breathe out negativity; breathe in health, breathe out disease. I can't seem to focus on one combination because there are so many things I want to be and so many I want to expel. In and out, in and out; my mind is a jumble. For once, I leave Jeanine's class far more agitated than when I arrived. I guess it's not a good idea to try too hard to get rid of stress— this just creates, no surprise here—more freaking stress!

After class, I'm determined to stay up at least until the kids turn in; Sam and Ben are leaving for a weekend trip with the high school band tomorrow. Lately, I've been in bed long before them, and I'm missing half the "fun" of having teenagers—listening to their music (Ben loves Led Zeppelin and Hendrix, groups I adored at his age), prodding them to do their homework, fixing a midnight snack. These days, I close my door at ten and crawl under my blankets, burrowing in with a book, and turning off the light by 10:30. I think of an opera singer warming up: "Mi, mi, mi, mi, mi!" (though Mitch says unlike the cartoon characters, real singers sound more like "meh, meh, meh"). In any case, I'm tired of me, me, me, tired of thinking about whether I'm doing everything right for my health. I'm tired of thinking, period. Maybe radiation *has* worn me down.

On this lovely spring Sunday Mitch is playing a concert in celebration of Mozart's 250th birthday held in a dusty but impressive mansion on the campus of a nearby college. Imagine being two hundred and fifty years old. I wonder where Mozart is now; if one buys into the reincarnation theory he could be a guitarist in a rock group like AudioSlave.

I sit in the back of the room since I haven't purchased a ticket (another perk of a musician's wife), and decide that instead of thinking about whether Mitch has tied his hair back properly, or whether his reed sounds harsh, or whether the young violinist seems to be making eyes at him, I am going to do one thing only: I am going to listen to the music with all my heart.

With my eyes closed, I focus on the sound of Mozart's Clarinet Quintet K. 581 in A Major, which quite possibly is the most beautiful piece ever written (of course, in my family, we're partial to clarinet selections). Still, there's nothing quite like Mozart, and as I follow the notes I realize that listening to music in this way is really a kind of meditation. If you experience the music note to note it's almost like a *walking* meditation; you just go with the music wherever it leads, and everything else seems to fall away. Halfway through the piece, I can't help thinking that this is the best I've ever heard my husband play.

I squint my eyes and peek at him; swaying slightly, looking so debonair in his black shirt and slacks (no tuxes at this event), with his silvery ponytail glimmering in the sunlight that filters through the ceiling to floor windows. I'm overcome by my love for him (and of course, for the music). One of the most effective ways to fall in love with your spouse again is to watch him work. No matter what your mate does for a living (unless, perhaps, if he's a mortician?) it always seems to me that work brings love to the surface. On the few occasions in the past when I've considered leaving Mitch, I've always known that if I ever heard a clarinet played beautifully (or even horribly!) anywhere I fled I'd regret my decision and have to turn back.

But maybe it's just the Mozart; a woman two seats ahead of me is amorously rubbing her husband's neck.

After the final piece I sidle up to Mitch. I don't usually say much about his performances because one comment will lead to twenty questions about reeds and tone, and barrels and mouthpieces. "You played great!" is about all I usually utter, which invariably leads to "in the second movement, did you notice the phrasing...did my tone sound dark..."

Today, however, at the end of the program I throw my arms around him and gush, "You've never played so beautifully! I've never heard the Mozart clarinet quintet sound so magical."

Instead of asking me a million questions or berating his equipment, Mitch looks softly into my eyes. "You noticed," he answers.

Either my husband is at the pinnacle of his career, or I'm finally learning how to really listen to music. Maybe both.

∞

On my way to radiation today, I glance into a room where a small woman rests on an examining table. She wears a kerchief on her head, and she's the color of ice; she must weigh all of eighty pounds. In that one quick glance, I can't tell if she's forty or ninety, but she has the appearance of a woman defeated by cancer, just biding her time. I feel a tug deep in my heart as I pass swiftly by, wishing I hadn't looked in. The simultaneous frailty and strength of the human condition are just so hard to fathom.

I sit in the waiting room, trying to erase the vision from my mind. As if in answer, a woman approaches the desk; she's tall, with very short black hair—so short that one knows she's been through chemo. She's wearing high-heeled sandals, scores of rings and bracelets, and her violet eyes are ringed with black liner. She takes a seat opposite me, and within moments we're in conversation. It turns out she's a poet, and she confides that she prefers to write about love rather than sorrow. "From the instant I found I had cancer," she says, "I decided that dying was not an option. I would do whatever I must to stay alive."

I'm called away for my treatment, but as I leave I wish her luck. I almost wish this were not my last day, and I could get to know her.

Almost, I said. Inside the treatment room, Denise is whistling and cheerful. "Your last day!" she smiles, moving me into position. "For you!"

She places a gift in my hands—a pair of beautiful, green fuzzy socks stenciled with butterflies. I gulp back tears as I thank her. I've never even mentioned my—or my mother's—relationship with the lovely papillon!

I hold still on my side while the machine clicks on for the very last time, and when Denise comes back to collect me, I give her a hug. I'm going to miss this pregnant lady!

At home, I serve dinner, and then step out for a walk. Outside, the sun is just setting and the sky is a muted pink. I walk past rabbits, mockingbirds, and robins, winding through the neighborhood onto a quiet street where few cars pass, thinking all the while of how grateful I am that radiation is over, of how lucky I am to have Jill in my life, of how much love I've been finding everywhere. I'm like GW with his "political capital," only mine is love capital, payback time for all my years of devotion to my mother, my family, my friends. Who gets fuzzy socks from their radiation therapist? With butterflies, no less. It almost seems as if the universe is responding to my deepest longings. Jill always says she just "puts it out there" and what she needs comes back like a boomerang. I've never bought into this kind of stuff in the past, but experiencing is believing. Maybe it was always there, and I just wasn't paying attention. Or perhaps things actually happen because we want and will them to. Perhaps a life can become filled with goodness because goodness is envisioned. Some would say I haven't been very lucky, getting breast cancer and all. But I feel luckier than I ever have. It's almost as if I was looking at life through a dusty window; now I've blown and rubbed on the pane, and suddenly a lustrous sunrise has come into view.

As I'm walking, my cell phone rings and I snatch it out of my pack, expecting one of the kids to be on the line. It's Evelyn, the bassoonist, looking for Mitch. She doesn't know that Mitch and I have recently switched phones. As soon as she hears my voice, she congratulates me on my completion of radiation; apparently, my husband has been keeping her apprised of my progress. "You're a warrior now," Evelyn says.

When I get home, I remember that a package has arrived in the mail from Mitch; he's ordered me a surprise from a woman we know in upstate New York who sells exquisite jewelry, and though he's working tonight, I plan to open the gift now that my treatments have come to their grand finale.

I sit at the dining room table and pull open the package.

Inside is a stunning amber amulet on a silver chain.

I step up to the mirror and fasten the clasp. The amber piece—about the size of a quarter—lands squarely on the uppermost of the seven tiny blue tattoos that encircle my breast, the one little blue speck that can be seen by the naked eye when I'm wearing a scooped neck.

A perfect fit.

∞

In yoga today, Jill instructs us to ease into our Headstands, stopping in a little pod before we go all the way up. The only way I have ever achieved a Headstand is by energetically flinging my feet against the wall. Today, I give the slow motion approach a try, and I do manage a pod for an instant. "That's enough," I tell Jill, "now I'm flinging my legs up."

Jill laughs, "You can do whatever you want!"

While we're in our pose, Jill says we should try to find the stillness within. "Remember," she says, "it's the chatter and noise that make that stillness so sacred."

After class, I find Sam in the kitchen, and I bring up the dicey subject of the prom. He's been debating whether to take Gretchen; after all, she's found a new boyfriend from another school, and it's just some sort of archaic sense of chivalry that's keeping Sam to his promise. Since Gretchen is only a junior, she can't attend without him.

I impart some yogic wisdom. "Just listen to your heart," I advise. "It will tell you what to do."

"My heart says to get the hell away from her!" Sam snaps.

Hopefully, time and the girls at Carnegie Mellon will ease his pain.

∞

Beth has the day off from her nursing job; to celebrate the

conclusion of my radiation and her birthday, as well as this beautiful May afternoon, we go out to lunch and then for a walk in the park. Oddly enough, as we're strolling around the pond, we see a woodchuck—in a small tree. The animal sways the top branches, then clambers down and scurries off through the grass. Beth and I are spellbound. In our fifty-three years, we've seen plenty of woodchucks (my father always called them "whistle-pigs") but never in a tree. I guess there's always room in life for something new.

When we finish our walk, I drop Beth home. "Just wait here a minute; I have something for you," she instructs. In a few moments, she emerges from her apartment with a plant I don't recognize. "Your end-of-radiation present. It's a butterfly plant!"

I've never heard of such a thing, but later, when I check online, I discover that not only is it not unusual for woodchucks to climb trees, but also that a plant called the butterfly plant, or butterfly weed, is quite common. Its tall stalk will eventually offer bright orange blossoms that will attract butterflies to my garden, or so the Internet claims.

"Just wondering," I ask Beth, after thanking her profusely. "Is there a reason why you chose a *butterfly* plant in particular?"

"I was looking for a bleeding heart, but I couldn't find one. So I got this instead. Anyway, I know you like butterflies."

"Actually, my mother was really fond of butterflies. And they seem to be turning up everywhere lately." I don't even mention the butterfly candle that I received yesterday as recompense for a talk on motherhood I gave at a local school.

Beth smiles, meeting my gaze with her large blue eyes. "Do you think Virginia is sending you a message, or is it just coincidence?"

I'm surprised that Beth—a born again Christian—is even asking that question!

∞

I'm dreading my visit to the oncologist today; whenever I think of going to what I call the "cancer circus" I feel frail again. Once you have breast cancer, you're watched carefully for several years with follow-ups to the oncologist and surgeon scheduled every few months.

I call it a circus—not to demean the patients, of whom I am one—but because twelve doctors share the same office, and there are literally fifty people in the outer waiting room, and that's not counting those in the inner waiting and treatment areas. Although I feel less intimidated than I did at my first visit, it's still a scary place: think dentist's office, and then multiply by a hundred. At the radiation treatment center, patients were scheduled in small groups, and only a few doctors were attending. Here, there's a long line at the check-in desk, as if we're all waiting for lattes and donuts.

I locate an empty seat, and bury myself in a novel, but I'm surrounded by pale-faced women in kerchiefs, patients in wheelchairs, and quite a few people who look perfectly healthy, though I suspect they are not. I glance at my watch; I've been here an hour already, and all they've done is take my blood and vitals. Ben and Sam are home from school by now, and I'm not there to ask how their day has gone. Of course, my kids aren't babies, and it's reasonable to expect them to fend for themselves while I go to the doctor. It's just that after six weeks of radiation, I want to be home again after school. I don't want to be anywhere near this hospital.

I'm ushered to an inner office where I wait another ten minutes, then to an examining room. I try to read, but in my distracted state I can't help wondering what in the hell I'll do if I have a recurrence of this dreaded disease. I'm fretting, too, that Dr. B may be preoccupied or unfriendly, though he wasn't that way before. Bottom line: I just don't want to be here.

I close my book and decide to alter my thoughts: there's no reason to sit here in a funk, expecting the worst. I remember a quote from the Indian mystic Kabir I recently came across: "... just throw away all thoughts of imaginary things, and stand firm in that which you are." *That which you are.*

I begin to consider how lucky I am to have a hospital so near my home where they seem to know what they're doing. I recall how much I adored Dr. B the last time I saw him, how gentle and funny he was. (I liked the way he noted the date of my telltale mammogram, commenting dryly that my holiday season must have been "real jolly.") I think about how grateful I am that I didn't have to do chemo, about how kind Denise and the others were at radiation, about how wonderful it is to know it's spring and I'm sitting here alive, looking forward to summer.

Dr. B strides into the room accompanied by a tall, smiling nurse. Granted, he doesn't waste time, glancing at my chart, asking me a few questions, but his startling blue eyes are not afraid to meet mine, and he gently touches my arm and tells me to call him if I experience any side effects from the hormone therapy pill I'm taking. He has an expression of abiding alertness, and I can only conclude that an oncologist must be living at the height of mindfulness. Here is a man who has devoted his life to paying attention to others, others, others, one by one, all day long, hour after hour, putting the puzzle pieces of all those blood tests, scans, and symptoms together time and time again, delivering bad news, delivering hope, offering solutions, offering knowledge. The man *has* to be living in the moment, because that is the only way he could do this job and not go stark raving mad.

My complaints fade away, my fear recedes, and one word once again comes to the forefront of my mind: gratitude. I'm tempted to squeeze his hand.

At class this evening Jeanine reminds us that the darkness, the fear, the difficult parts of life deserve mindfulness, just as do the lighter parts of life, and it occurs to me that even in a room filled with cancer patients, so many faces hold beauty and strength. I think back to a couple I saw this afternoon; a ruddy, middle-aged man with a baseball cap and faded jeans, grasping the small, white hand of his wife. She was bald from chemo, dressed in baggy sweats and sneakers. They could have chosen to sit farther apart, or to bury their faces in a newspaper. Instead, as husband and wife, they kept their connection, their hands entwined, gripping one another during the hours they sat in the waiting room. Maybe they were thinking about how afraid they were, or worrying about what would happen when they got inside the office. Or, maybe they were realizing how lucky they were to have each other's hand to hold; maybe they were savoring one another's touch.

Tonight, in a drenching, windy rain, our apple tree crashes to the ground and can't be resurrected. So much for symbolism, I do hope.

I awaken to the sound of a meowing cat. Funny, because I've been dreaming about a book my mother used to read to me when I was a child, a book called *Big Little Kitty*, though it takes me a few foggy moments to remember the title. The cat in the book, as I recall, was named Muffin.

When I look out the window I'm expecting to see that cute little scotch-colored kitten on my deck, but instead there's an old, fat black cat sitting next to the felled apple tree, howling away.

I decide to Google *Big Little Kitty* when I come downstairs, and sure enough there's a first edition copy for sale on EBay, the only reference to the book I can find online. My memory has served me correctly; according to the description, the cat's name is Muffin, and she runs away from home and gets into all kinds of mischief. The book was published in 1953, the year I was born, and I probably haven't thought of it since I was six or seven.

When I glance up from my computer again, the black cat has left and a scotch-colored cat is stretched out on the deck. Muffin all grown up? My yard has never before been such a haven for felines.

Another spooky thing has recently occurred in my yard. The butterfly plant has bloomed—not into little orange blossoms as expected, but into beautiful translucent blue flowers, with petals the precise size and shape of butterfly wings, and delicate curled antennae. Surely this is no weed, and I can't find it anywhere online.

Out of curiosity, I returned to the shop where Beth made the purchase, but none of the attendants remembered it, or knew its name, and there were no other plants like it anywhere in the store. I carried a blossoming sprig to several other nurseries, but no one could make an identification.

"Hmm, I've never seen the likes of this!" one aging horticulturalist told me, scratching her head. "But I do believe it's some kind of annual—it won't be back next year."

I've convinced Mitch to come along to a "restorative" yoga class; it's Mother's Day and Natalie has encouraged us to bring our husbands or older children. Jill has set out mats, bolsters, weights and eye pillows and about fifteen of us hunker down (yes, a few other husbands grudgingly come along) while she guides us through the various resting positions. It feels somewhat strange to have Mitch in the class, but only because I usually take yoga seriously and with my husband here I'm tempted to fool around. Our fingers touch as we move into a pose on our backs side by side, and Mitch slyly holds a long slim bolster erect to tease me. We're laughing aloud but no one seems to mind.

The mood turns more somber when Jill tells us to close our eyes and imagine our mother, to think of her smile, her touch, or the way she hugs us. Of course, I think about the fact that I haven't been hugged by my mom in almost five years, but I'm able to remember her smile and touch without crying; I'm actually able to happily recall her sweetness and generosity.

On our way out, I ask Mitch how he liked the session.

"I don't need help relaxing; *I* can relax anytime I want. But I can see the value for a person like *you*."

"A person who's uptight and can't keep her mind from spinning?"

"Exactly. But I'm surprised you didn't cry when your teacher started in about mothers," he observes.

That surprised me, too. Yet on the other hand, this is exactly what I've been striving for—the ability to feel an emotion without being destroyed by it, the ability to see the fear and anguish coming, and *choose* to go another way, to be the guide and healer of my own thoughts, and not a person who follows myself into the darkness at every opportunity. No, I'm not so surprised after all.

At home, the boys have made me a Mother's Day brunch. The French toast is oddly salty, and the omelet tastes like cinnamon as if they've reversed their spices, but I eat every bite. Ben has prepared a fruit salad, and Sam is washing up the dishes. Aaron makes me a cup of tea. Heavenly.

Later, Aaron and Ben head for the mall, and Sam, Mitch and I take a hike at a local nature center. We can't help remembering that this is the very trail Sam first really walked on—taking off down the winding path through the woods as a curious toddler. He's still ahead of us, pointing out chipmunks and birds, but he's quite a bit taller. He turns to me and holds *my* hand as we hop across the slippery rocks in the stream.

We reconnect with our other children for dinner at a Chinese restaurant. As "Circle of Life" plays in the background, Ben turns to me and whispers, "You're not getting all choked up now, are you?" He's a very perceptive kid. And he's right, that song just always does it to me, especially now.

I step outside when we get home and survey the apple tree, which is on its side, its branches grazing our blackberry patch. Some might question why we allow an immense blackberry patch to meander across the yard's center, nearly blocking access to our garage. But to taste the pies I bake in July or to watch three boys in the heat of summer wearing winter gloves as they pluck the juicy berries from the thorns and pop them into their mouths is to know the answer.

I try to look at the tree's demise positively; there will be more sun on the deck. I can plant wildflowers and tomatoes. I can buy a new tree, maybe a pink dogwood or a thundercloud plum. I try to envision the possibilities, and I know what Jill would say: "This is life. This is change." Yes, there's a huge empty hole where the apple tree stood. Now, how can I fill it?

I'm determined to purchase a new tree, so Mitch and I spend the morning at a vast local nursery, contemplating the dogwoods, plum trees and cherries. He can't understand my hurry; it's not very "Zen" of me, he says. And I can't really understand it, either; all I know is I miss the graceful arms of my apple tree over my deck, and I want that empty space to be filled.

After an hour or so of debate, we settle on a plum tree. The owner of the nursery assures me that I'd be hard-pressed to kill this sturdy variety, but the purple-pink blossoms are the real clincher; my apple tree had the sweetest pink blossoms, and I'd like to gaze out my window next spring and see those colors again.

We drive home with the six-foot Vesuvius Plum in our van. It just fits—the pot is at the very back and the weightless, red leaves are grazing our heads. It's an awesome feeling to give a tree a lift.

∞

I tell Jill about the apple tree today, and she has a weird reaction.

"Good!" she cries. "The new tree is your new life; transformed and cancer-free." Apparently, while I've been identifying with the apple tree, Jill's interpretation is that it symbolized my old life and the cancer. I guess you can make a symbol out of anything you want, and you can interpret it to mean whatever you want, too. It figures that Jill would have a positive reaction while I see the tree's demise as an evil omen. I guess I still need to work on my outlook.

We focus on Warrior Three today, which requires a good bit of core strength. You stand on one leg with the other lifted behind and bend forward, reaching your arms straight ahead. Jill says to think of our chakras—to concentrate on our power, our center of strength, which is represented by yellow. I think of the yellow irises that were in my garden this morning when I stepped out to come to class. Yesterday their buds were folded and today they're bright and full. I manage to hold the pose without toppling over.

"When you can walk through your fears, that is courage," Jill says out of the blue. I close my eyes and envision a path with clouds of fear on either side; I see myself walking through the center, forging ahead, battling away my negative thoughts like Papageno in The Magic Flute.

As always, I wonder how Jill knows so much about what goes on in our hearts and minds. But we all have fears, and we all need to be strong to get past them.

∞

I have a very busy day—three deadlines for the local parenting newspaper, paying bills, shopping, cooking. When I leave all my papers sitting on the dining room table and head out the door, Mitch asks me if I really "need" to go to yoga tonight. I hesitate, but only for a moment, before I answer yes and drive off.

It's a good thing I've come, because Jeanine is focused tonight on something she calls "non-doing." In my day, we used to call this kicking back, lolling around, or to put it bluntly, fucking off. How amazing that I am paying sixteen dollars a class to fuck off, to sprawl on my back, with my arms outstretched, listening to tinkling piano music in the background. I could laze around on my own carpet, after all; I could put on an airy New Age CD and fuck off at my own leisure.

Yet I know I wouldn't do that, and so I'd pay just about any amount of money to come to Jeanine's class. Her melodic voice, calling out directions to stretch this limb or that, slips in and out of the music. She brings us blankets and bolsters and helps us position for the greatest comfort. We bend into Child's pose over bolsters and she tiptoes around the room, giving massages.

Jeanine talks about how important it is to make time for "non-doing" in our days. I used to think being busy was the key to everything—and especially to overcoming fear or grief. Common advice is to keep occupied after a death; busyness is supposed to ward off disturbing thoughts, sort of the way garlic repels vampires.

But there's a difference between mindless busyness (or escapism) and filling your days with meaningful activities. And there's a difference between fucking off and non-doing. Damned if I can *explain* the difference, but trust me on this.

∞

Tonight is the Spring Concert—the last spring concert that Sam will ever play. I'm not the only one cognizant of this fact; most of the mothers of seniors are wiping tears from their eyes, and the senior girls in the band (why is it always the girls?) are visibly choking back tears all throughout the concert.

Sam is on French horn tonight, and Ben is playing alto saxophone. After years of attending these concerts, I've figured out exactly where to sit so I can see my children, but tonight I'm also positioned so that I can clearly see Gino, who plays the trombone. As his fingers grasp the instrument's golden slide, I think about what a beautiful boy he is, so full of life and vitality, his hair grown in black and thick now that his chemo is over, his dark eyes sparkling. Like Sam, he'll be going off to college in the fall.

Amazingly, I'm not overcome by sadness as I watch our seniors play their last spring concert; I'm filled with anticipation about what life will hold for these kids.

I email Jill to ask if she can recommend a book on the yoga sutras. When I take one out from the library it expires before I can plow through it, so I'm determined to buy a copy of my own that I can take my time reading. She emails back that a yogi who wrote such a book is speaking "today" at the other yoga center where she also teaches, and I am welcome to come.

It's a beautiful late May Sunday morning and I can think of several or more reasons why I don't want to spend my afternoon sitting on the floor of a studio with some yogi guru, but after a walk with Mitch I decide that since Jill has recommended this guy, I should attend. After all, why did I email her willy-nilly on the very day a sutra expert is speaking? Why, *indeed.*

When we arrive, the owner of the center begins chanting in Sanskrit. I chime in with the others, though we could be chanting

"Oh, what a goose I am" for all I know. She then introduces the speaker, who makes himself comfy in a large, over-stuffed chair while we gather round on little pillow-seats scattered on the hardwood floor. The reverend (who knows what *kind* of reverend?) is a hefty man with a glowing gray beard. I long for the sunshine outside; this guru worship smacks of ritualistic cultism, if you ask me.

As the man begins to lecture, I suspect that maybe the guy was an English major; he sounds like a lot of college professors I once knew, and he has a certain confidence—as if he could talk circles around us all forever. He takes questions from the audience, and I'm reminded even more of a college lecture hall. I can't figure out why all these middle-aged moms are giving up their Sunday afternoon to sit with their legs crossed and cramping, listening to some yogi ramble on about the meaning of life.

I like the reverend's analogies, though, and I'm attracted to the clownish twinkle in his eye. He doesn't take himself too seriously, even though he's barefoot and wearing white. He's talking about the usual yogi topics: what makes us happy (not TVs, cars, etcetera), how we need to fill our lives with goodness to flush out the bad stuff, how each situation is an opportunity for growth, cancer. Wait a minute; this dude is talking about cancer!

I lean forward, trying to figure out how he's arrived at this subject. Apparently, one of the women has asked what to do if something tragic happens to you, and the yogi is using cancer as an example. He tells a story of three dolls—a glass doll, a wooden doll, and a bronze doll—all hit by the same hammer. The glass doll, fragile and without support, shatters; the wooden doll, in denial with her head in the sand, makes a thud, but the bronze doll—the yogini—rings like a bell, letting her best self shine.

I think about my breakfast out with Mitch this morning, and of how he said that I'm better since the cancer. My body looks and feels better than ever; my spirit feels more at peace.

We can all choose, this yogi says, our response to the pain in life, the pain that is inevitable for everyone. "And why," he asks, "should we not believe that death itself is the most beautiful thing?"

I have tears in my eyes when I leave, carrying a copy of the guru's book, a gift from Jill. Foiled again—my skepticism vanquished by wonder.

Tonight, as I fall asleep, I imagine that there might be an afterlife, and I wish that my mother would send me a message. I gaze at my bedroom window, noticing the shadows of our pine tree, fluttering against the curtains, filtered through a distant light. With a wind blowing strong even in the warm spring air, the shadows resemble dozens of butterflies. I rise up on my elbow and reach for my glasses. With my glasses on, I'll be able to see clearly, and I will laugh at myself. But when I put them on my eyes, the shadows look even *more* distinctly like butterflies, dancing joyfully in the night.

Not surprisingly, Jill talks about our outing in class today. She retells the story of the glass doll, and as I listen, I wonder how many women here really "get" it. I know it wouldn't have resounded in quite the same way for me before my diagnosis. But now, I want to be that bronze yogini, ringing more beautifully than ever before.

Later, I con Mitch into helping me make my breast mold for the traveling sculpture exhibit, even though I'm worried that Sam or Ben will pop in on us. They'd probably be scarred for life if they were to see their mother, naked from the waist up, being painted with purple goo by their father. More likely, our mailman will have a stroke if he peers into the window by the doorway.

Nevertheless, we spread out our materials on the kitchen

table and Mitch mixes and stirs, then paints my breast with the thick purple liquid, which is then covered with strips of wet gauze. The instructions say to stand still for twenty minutes while it dries, and of course, I can't help thinking of that "other" mold while I'm motionless. Mitch switches on the TV for me, and I distract myself with Tony Danza's talk show (I once had a horrific crush on the man). I glance down at my breasts; the left one looks just as before, the right is covered with the cast, which is strangely warm to the touch. Maybe life is just a weak imitation of art instead of vice versa. Anyway, I can see Tony but it's a damn good thing he can't see me.

After what seems an eternity, the cast is dry, and Mitch gently tugs it off my breast. Before we place it in a box to be mailed to the sculptress, I ask him to take a photo of me holding it against my body. I put my shirt back on and pose with the plaster breast. I suppose the image would be more dramatic if I posed naked, but I'm not that comfy in front of the camera. I'm just a breast cancer survivor mom who wants a picture to remember making my mold. *Just?* I'm tempted to feel self-pity when I peer at my small deformity, but then I remember that the exhibit is really about our power and strength. Mitch snaps my picture, though I'm not sure he understands why I want one. To me, it seems like some kind of talisman; the sculpted breast embodies my pain and disease, which I'm sending off to join a traveling exhibit. My real breast can now go back to being "her old self."

In the afternoon, Mitch is at a ballet rehearsal so after working on my newspaper articles, I take a walk. I walk almost every day now, or practice yoga. I walk for two reasons: my health and my peace of mind. I find that when I walk everything is sharper and brighter than it has ever been, even on a drab, rainy day. On a sunny day like today, the pink of a rhododendron or the perfume of a wild rose bush is astonishing. I am learning to live fully in each moment; like the guru said, I want to fill my life with beautiful thoughts, and flush out the rest.

Tonight, we attend the National Honor Society inductions. Last year, even though he would have been inducted, Gino was unable to make it because he was in the midst of his health crisis. This year, wearing his golden robe, he sits next to Sam on the stage; they are passing the torch to the incoming inductees. When Sam turns and lights Gino's candle with his own it feels as if they've made the entire auditorium glow. This is not just the light of knowledge; this is also the light of love.

Today, Jill leads us in a white light meditation, asking us to envision a healing, white light traveling through our bodies. We sit silently as she guides us visually from our toes to our head. Even though I'm a personal fan of white light, I still wonder if any of this hocus-pocus really works. It would be so wonderful if we could heal the whole world with our thoughts.

Of course, that's not possible. But I do believe we can make ourselves sick by cluttering up our minds with negativity. Maybe cancer comes from other things—drinking too much wine, eating red meat, inhaling toxins, whatever—but I've come to believe that our thinking does have an impact on the outcome. And even if positive thoughts don't actually cure, they certainly help us to enjoy and appreciate the days and moments we do have. The end of school is like a crescendo; there is so much happening in the next few weeks, mostly fun and pleasant, like the prom and various celebratory awards dinners. I'm really looking forward to so many occasions. I remember when Aaron graduated—every last event brought me to tears. But now, I'm different. I am finally beginning to believe in the concept that change need not be battled; it can be embraced. And I do feel joy as I anticipate the future; after all, I still have Ben's graduation to look forward to. I can imagine Ben stepping up to get his diploma, following in his brothers' steps, yet listening to his own calling, whether that may be writing, computers, or playing guitar in a heavy metal band.

Just the other day, I asked Mitch why musical terms are necessary. Why not say, "slow down" instead of adagio? Why not say "fast" instead of allegro? The book I'm now reading on the yoga sutras prompted this; the author uses Sanskrit phrases and with all those unfamiliar words, I feel as if I'm reading Chaucer for the first time. But I can't find a better word for "vritti," the Sanskrit term for the way our thoughts rush to tangle in intricate webs. And I can't find a better word for this crescendo at the end of Sam's senior year. In truth, I can't really find a better word than crescendo for the way I feel about living in general these days, as if my whole past has been building up to this time when I finally appreciate the beauty and depth of now.

At Jeanine's class tonight, a fellow student inquires whether my radiation is over. When I say yes she congratulates me and asks what I'm doing these days. I don't think I'll ever respond "nothing" or "oh, not much" to that question ever again.

"Living my life fully," I answer. Only in yoga class can you get away with a comeback like that. If I'd been at a Manhattan cocktail party I'd have been booted out on my ass.

The prom is tonight, and Sam is in a funk because Gretchen didn't even speak to him today at school. As we drive to pick up her corsage I advise, "Just have fun with your friends; after tonight, you won't have to hang out with Gretchen again if she makes you uncomfortable!"

No response, and I can tell he doesn't want to talk about it, but as we exit the car at the florist's I add, "Why don't we change the lavender and white flowers we've ordered to something more garish that won't match her gown? How about those Saint Patty's Day carnations with the green trim?"

Sam laughs, and nods toward some dandelions growing in the cracks of the sidewalk. "These would do," he says.

Inside the florist's shop, however, he's upset that the wrist corsage we've ordered has pink instead of white sweetheart roses, and his boutonnière is pink as well, instead of purple. He asks the shopkeeper to change the flowers, so we wait until she makes the adjustments. Clearly, he's not a punishing sort of boy; he wants Gretchen's flowers to properly match her dress even though she's dropped him.

At five, the kids all gather at one of the girl's homes, along with the paparazzi parents. I bring along my camera, and the teens pose while we all take pictures. The boys look dashing in their tuxedos; Sam's is black (and free—his musician father's, lucky boy), with a rented lavender vest and tie to match Gretchen's dress. The girls are adorned in pastel, full-length gowns, many with cleavages showing. First we take couples, then Sam and Gino pose with the other boys, and the girls gather for their group portraits. The parents seem to be having almost as much fun as the kids.

Just before the limo is set to take off, Sam steps away from his friends, motioning for my camera. He hands it to Mitch and then pulls me toward him. "Take our picture?" he asks his dad.

I'm touched, and surprised; I don't know too many teenaged boys who would think of this on their own. We put our arms around each other's waists, and Mitch clicks the shutter. This is a picture I'll want to keep in my heart.

∞

I'm in a foul mood today because I'm missing Jill's class due to a follow-up visit with the urologist, whose office is located at the hospital. My bladder seems to have calmed down (the combination of the cystoscopy procedure itself and my new alcohol-free diet, perhaps), but the doctor also admits that stress may have caused the flare-up. In any case, I'm dismissed with a clean slate, though I can't help thinking back to how often patients are told everything's fine when somewhere in the body there's cancer already brewing. (My mother was given a clean bill of health by a doctor and advised to go off with me on a nice, relaxing vacation two weeks before she died.) No doubt these negative thoughts are intensified when the elevator stops at the fourth floor—home to the cancer circus—on the way to the lobby. Sure enough, there's the line of patients waiting to be processed. I'm grateful that I don't have to go *there* today.

I step out into the cavernous garage, feeling, as Ben says, as if I "totally own" this hospital now. This looming, construction-laden place used to intimidate the hell out of me. Not any more. After thirty-three trips to radiation oncology, and countless doctor visits, I even know how to brazenly sneak beneath the "Do Not Enter" signs in the bustling parking garage to hunt down the hidden spots that are always empty. I know the winding path to the various medical wings, and which elevators to take. I even know where to get an awesome cup of coffee. Yes, like it or not, I totally *own* this place.

When I arrive home, Jill phones. "Where have you been?" she asks. "Natalie and I were concerned because you didn't show up for class."

"Not to worry. Just a routine check-up."

It's so unlike her to fret, but I'm such a fixture there now that my absence is noticed; I realize that cancer is not only *my* journey, it's something that, through me, has also touched my teachers, family, and friends. The cancer "victim" or "survivor" feels alone in many ways, but the bottom line is that this disease scares the shit out of *everyone*.

I step out onto my deck tonight and whisper pleasantries to my new plum tree. I trickle-water it each night, hoping it will grow and blossom. A bright, male cardinal is singing above me, and the yard is awash with green leaves and colorful flowers; a four-foot tall Dame's Rocket—in full purple bloom—has sprouted in my garden out of nowhere, right next to the mysterious "butterfly" plant. Standing here, in the warm spring air, I realize that there's no point in hoping for that pot at the *end* of the rainbow. The whole damn rainbow itself *is* the pot of gold.

Destination: Here

I'm missing Jill's class again; this time it's my follow up with the radiation oncologist. Dr. G examines my skin and proclaims, "You look fine. Just stay healthy!" I ask her about a few aches and pains, but she says they don't sound serious. I wonder if I'll ever get over the fear that every twinge is cancer.

On the way out I search for Denise, my radiation therapist. We hug in the hallway, and she tells me I look great. She looks great, too—three weeks have made a difference in her pregnancy and her belly is round and full. In a few more months she'll be starting her own unique journey with a new baby.

As we turn and head down the hall, Mitch asks, "Are you getting emotional?" (After nearly twenty-nine years of marriage the man has figured out that I'll cry at just about anything, particularly good-byes.) Truth be known, I *do* feel saddened saying a final farewell to Dr. G and Denise, but I'll be happy if I never have to see this wing of the hospital again. Today, instead of crying, I skip down the hall away from this place like a blissful lunatic.

∞

Jill calls and asks, "Would you like to go with me to a restorative yoga class later? It's at a center I used to frequent when I first started practicing. My treat!"

"Sure," I say. "I'm always open to new possibilities these days." Besides, I missed Jill's class yesterday, and I'd like to see her.

We meet at the yoga studio, a narrow space connected to a manicurist's shop; indeed, the yoga instructor herself turns out to be the manicurist. She's a small yogini with a tiny waist and delicate features, but I can immediately tell that when it comes to yoga, the woman means business. Much to my surprise, this yoga class is run in the Iyengar style, a method which is apparently very meticulous about the tiniest movements. We bend over at the waist, attached with belts to a pole in the center of the room; we stretch our legs with belts, we turn our torsos, while the instructor places beanbag weights on our arms and legs. I sense disapproval when I fail to position my arms correctly, but when I smile warmly, the instructor warms in return.

Jill appears to be enjoying herself. It's unusual to practice side by side; I'm used to her being the teacher, of course. Although I appreciate this new instructor's knowledge, I realize that Jill's patient teaching style is much better suited to the way I learn. It seems to me that yoga should seep into one's soul and bones over time. The belt and weight routine seems a bit heavy-handed to me, though the "seven-blanket Savasana," which involves building a comfy mound to rest upon, is pure heaven.

As we leave, Jill explains to me that the Iyengar method is quite different than her Vinyasa approach, and I realize once again that even within the world of yoga, there are many paths one can follow. I'm still on the beginner's trail, but if one chooses, one can veer off onto the expert slopes, where the teachers are more demanding, the poses more precise, and the level of competition (in a practice which supposedly involves no competition) more intense. Sometimes I overhear students talking about classes they've taken with various gurus— revered instructors the yogi supplicants trail to workshops and retreats all over the world. But that's not for me; for now, I'm quite content to sit on my mat a block from my home. In yoga, you really don't need to go very far to travel into the universe, and deep into the soul.

After the session we linger in the parking lot, just chatting. "What did you cover in class this morning?" I inquire.

"I opened by passing out a roll of toilet paper and asking each student to take as many squares as she liked. Some took one or two squares, but others grabbed a handful. Once the roll had been passed around the studio, I asked everyone to come up with one positive quality about herself for each square that she held in her hands."

"Hmm, that's interesting. How did it go?" I can imagine some of the power yoginis babbling on.

Jill smiles. "Well, several of the students were very upset, and didn't want to share even *one* attribute. It was surprising; some of the more proficient students were very reluctant! It's difficult for us to be positive and confident about ourselves."

I'm sorry I missed this class. A year ago I would have had trouble coming up with a word or two. No doubt words like "plump" or "incompetent" would have sprang to mind instantly. But now, I eagerly review the words I might have used: brave, healthy, powerful, strong, caring, kind...the list in my mind goes on and on. If I were in class today, I could have used up the whole damn roll of toilet paper (Mitch always marvels over the amount I use, anyway). Yoga has given me permission to think kindly of myself and to know my own power. I think of the Chinese fortune cookie's message I found after lunch: "You are the master of every situation." Yogini translation: "You *are* the mistress of your universe!"

∞

Back to Dr. L. This doctor thing is getting tiresome, but this is the last I will see of my surgeon for six months, assuming all goes well with my upcoming follow-up MRI and mammogram.

Dr. L goes over my chart, and then asks me to recline on the examining table. I know what's coming, and I can't help noticing the pounding of my own heart. Once again, her gentle fingers knead my breasts; as I was the very first time here, I am quiet and solemn. I don't want to distract my doctor from her work; I don't think I'll ever utter a word during a breast exam again. Perhaps my cancer couldn't have been detected by this kind of exam in its earliest stages, but I have a feeling that if Dr. L had been checking, it would have been found even sooner than it was. I find it astonishing that most breast lumps have been growing for years before they're discovered.

She smiles when the exam is complete. "Everything looks great. I'll see you in six months so call the office and make an appointment. I'll phone with your MRI results, of course."

"Will you call either way?"

"I will call either way."

"I'm so afraid, whenever I feel any little pain, that it's cancer again," I confide.

"That's perfectly normal," she says. "Just give yourself time."

I'm grateful that I've found a physician who seems to understand my feelings. And I know, from the way Dr. L follows up on every test and protocol, that she'll be watching me closely.

When I step out of her office, I look up at the sky. There's an enormous thundercloud forming to the right, and the rest of the sky ranges from dark gray to blue. I can smell the winsome wild roses tangled in the hedges; this, I suspect, would be the "aroma" of hope.

∞

Tomorrow is our 29th wedding anniversary. To jumpstart the celebration, we have a horrendous fight.

The festivities begin when I head outside with the electric hedge trimmers to cut back *our* wild rose bush, which has been expanding into the driveway so frenetically that it's now impossible to get in and out of the cars without appearing to have been scratched and mauled by wild animals. I've been promising Mitch for weeks I will trim the bush as soon as it's done blooming, and today, having observed that the tiny white petals have all fallen to the ground, I decide to follow through.

Mitch trails me into the drive, but after a few moments of watching me gingerly snip, he stalks out to the garage, returning with the heavy-duty pruning shears. I don't know why I'm relating to trees and bushes so personally lately, but as soon as I see my husband with this violent instrument I freak. "Leave that bush alone!" I order. "Back off, will you? *I'm* handling this!"

But he ignores me. Before I know it he's removed several of the interior canes, and within seconds, the full, glorious bush is reduced to a sniveling little clump. He's usurped my power over what I consider to be "my" rose bush. He has trimmed without my permission and approval, in what I consider to be a cruel and aggressive manner.

I toss my hedge trimmers on the ground, scream out a few unsavory expletives (loud enough to cause my new neighbors to slam shut their windows), and dash up to my bedroom to cry under my pillow. Twenty-nine years, indeed! How could I have lived with this man for a single *day*?

Obviously, I have not mastered the yogic principle of "nonattachment." I am utterly attached to rose bushes, plum and apple trees, my children, my house, my deceased parents, to my decaf coffee, my emerald earrings, to my collection of Jane

Austen books. I am attached to the sky, the moon, the grass, the sun, and to my right breast, as well! When Mitch trims my rose bush, I feel as if my happiness has been stolen, even though I know logically that the bush will grow back healthier than ever. Even though I understand that my happiness has nothing to do with rose bushes or any other external object. Yes, I know this, but it doesn't seem to matter.

At first.

After an hour of feeling sorry for myself, I emerge from my room. The boys are tiptoeing politely around the kitchen, fixing their own breakfasts, whispering to me that they're "on my side."

"I'm sorry," Mitch concedes, "but the bush will certainly grow back."

"Hmmf," I respond, but not unkindly. "I sure hope so."

In the past, I would have played my anger out for several days, possibly even for a week or more, but this time, I accept his apology and drive off to Jeanine's meditation circle. With my eyes closed in this silent, candle-lit room, I try to find forgiveness. "Forgive the person, even if you can't forgive the action," Jill has said. No, I can't help feeling attached and angry at times; but now I can get over it sooner and without the same degree of injury. I can sit here with my legs crossed and my fingers pressed together; I can empty my mind, feel my heart beat, follow my breath, and reach inside for peace.

Putting the rose bush incident behind us (though warning my husband not to lay a finger on my lilacs), we start the fifth of June, our anniversary day, by making love (after the kids have gone to school, of course) followed by a delicious lunch at a Lebanese restaurant. Afterwards, Mitch insists on going shopping to buy me a new bathing suit; the town pool has opened.

We drive to an inexpensive department store and I pull a few suits off the rack and head for the dressing room while Mitch waits outside. Although the first three suits are too revealing, they fit just fine. I decide on a slightly tamer, shimmering gold and brown number, totally unlike the blues and greens I usually choose. As I stand before the mirror checking the size, I'm amazed that I don't feel a hint of displeasure. This is the first year in decades that I can remember being satisfied with what I see. I am not overweight (though I'm not "thin"), my muscles are sculpted (though not pronounced), and though I am obviously not a youngster, I have a damn "good" body. I am a fifty-three-year-old yogini, and I look it. I would not recommend the cancer weight loss program to anyone (I'm sure the stress and worry of what I've gone through has helped me shed that final unwanted five pounds), but I *do* highly recommend the yogic menu for life: practicing the asanas and discovering one's own power can work wonders on a woman's figure.

I'm celebrating another anniversary this week: two years of practicing yoga. I can't even begin to measure the ways that I've changed.

Before class today, Jill gives me a present; a small, abalone butterfly pin, to mark the end of my treatments. She knows, of course, what butterflies mean to me. And she knows that when I wear this pin, I will think not only of my mother, but also of how Jill herself has helped me to change, of how she has guided me in my metamorphosis from a fearful, nervous, middle-aged mom, to a hopeful, strong, confident yogini. I joke with the kids now, calling myself "Swami Mommy." But the truth is, I do feel that I have gained much more wisdom in the past two years than in all the years before combined. Finally, I feel as if not only do I have questions, I have at least a few answers. Finally, I can re-direct my thoughts and calm my own fears; I can replace my negative chattering with positive observations; I can believe in myself.

Today, in class, Jill talks about how we can find what is sacred, what is meaningful, in every moment, and I realize that this is perhaps the most important message I have learned both from yoga, and from cancer. It's not just about recognizing how "precious" every moment is, or about "living for today." It's about finding the sacred center of now, and living there, moment to moment, always.

This morning, Jill asks us to move our mats across the room so we're facing the rising sun. Sun Salutations—first introduced hundreds of years ago— are traditionally practiced in the morning facing east, and since it's been raining for four days straight she apparently thinks this is a good time to do them. At first, I panic at the thought of moving my mat, but when I laugh aloud and voice my fear, several other yoginis admit they don't want to move, either. We're all accustomed to our "spots" but we obediently follow Jill's instructions.

Now we're facing the east wall of the room, and Jill, too, has moved her mat to a new location. "Think about the sun," she says. "Think about how it shines brilliantly even though we can't always see it, about how it gives us warmth, offering itself unconditionally."

To me, Jill is the sun personified—she's always encouraging and offering herself to her students, providing spiritual light and wisdom. With her shiny red hair and sparkling sky-blue eyes, she even *looks* a bit like the sun, today.

I adore the breathy energy of sun salutations, and even when Jill throws in a pose she calls Wild Thing, I give it a try. It's some kind of Side Plank, with one leg thrown askew, and a Back Bend incorporated. This sort of pose looks great on the cover of a yoga magazine, but when I attempt it I'm sure I resemble a critically wounded camel. That's okay—I'm laughing; I've moved my mat, and I'm trying. The rain continues to pour down outside.

In Savasana, I think about the idea of non-attachment. I raised my children in a style called "attachment parenting," which basically meant I was either holding, nursing, or sleeping with them 24 hours a day when they were babies (other than Aaron's first year, when I was still at the magazine). This was supposed to give them a firm, confident base so that when they grew up they'd be surefooted and independent. It only took Ben six years to wrench himself out of our bed, but who's counting. Anyway, he *has* become a confident kid. And Sam went all the way to England on his own at age fifteen. And Aaron—unafraid to get on a plane to Tokyo, ready to hunt down an apartment now and live on his own. It's hard to believe these kids are my offspring, but maybe I *have* succeeded in keeping my fears to myself. Of course, they have the advantage of a fearless father. The only thing that seems to have frightened Mitch was my illness, but he never let me know, and I wouldn't know now if Anneke hadn't spilled the beans about a heart-to-heart she had with him one night when I was out. I love the way my girlfriends corner my husband.

Maybe I've even succeeded in getting rid of some of my fears completely. I do feel ready to board an airplane again; I really want to take a trip with Mitch to Paris—and Italy sounds good, too. I even imagine us noshing on goat cheese and olives while lazing by the Mediterranean.

Before I settle in to sleep tonight, I read a few passages from *Autobiography of a Yogi*, the story of a singular Indian sage who came to America in the early 1900s. I'm amazed to find that Paramahansa Yogananda was not present at his mother's death—the woman he considered his "dearest friend on earth." But instead of flogging himself for the rest of his life, he thanked the "Intervening Hand" for His compassion. Yogananda believed that whenever someone he loved deeply passed away, God graciously *arranged for him to be absent* to spare him from pain.

I close the book and whisper, "Thank *you*, Yogananda." At last, I can forgive myself.

∞

Today I read in the newspaper of a woman who died after a thirteen-year battle with breast cancer. Imagine the courage and strength that woman must have had. Amidst her pain, I hope that she had blissful days; I hope that she lived those thirteen years to their fullest potential. I'm awed by what she must have endured.

When I check the mail today, I find a notice from my insurance company, informing me that they won't cover the three thousand dollar test my doctor ordered that determined the nature of my cancer and helped him decide on my treatment. The test is "experimental," they claim. I suspect that they just don't want to start paying for this test for everyone, even though in a portion of cases it can make the difference between chemo and no chemo. I guess they think that all cancer victims should go through chemo just for fun and frolic.

Tonight, at yoga, Jeanine plays Greek music on the CD player and we dance in a circle. We step and dip to the right, then to the left, then work in a Warrior One. We mirror each other's movements, and howl with laughter. I think of the Iyengar class I attended last week with Jill. My, what a difference! Jeanine is a rebel yogini, and she never judges our poses. The closest she ever comes is to call out, "Be playful! Have fun!"

I *am* having fun tonight, laughing and dancing. For a moment I feel guilty. Six months after my diagnosis I'm filled with joy. How is it that one woman had to battle for thirteen years?

In Savasana, Jeanine describes a trip to Greece. We imagine we sit by the ocean, bathed in a golden light. Her voice carries us far away, and yet I am deep within myself, in the place of my own that yoga has given to me.

∞

At the sports awards dinner, I am moved to tears. It all begins with three hours of speeches and a light dinner in our local meeting hall. I've never attended this annual event before, because, to be honest, my kids aren't exactly sports stars, and I'm not really keen on "sports people."

The speeches are long, but not exactly boring, because I do know many of these kids. Sam is here of course; he insisted on bowling and playing baseball this year. Plus he was the co-drum major of the band, dressed head to toe in a white uniform, which afforded him a certain panache at the football games. He's sitting on the other side of the vast, airy hall with his friends.

I'm judgmental when the evening begins and I wonder how I can live in a small town and be so out of touch with such a large portion of the populace. I've always looked down my nose at the coaches, too. They can't be *real* teachers, I've always thought, if all they do is coach sports. Of course, most of them do teach other subjects. If you consider keyboarding or phys ed to be "subjects."

When I see how much they love the kids, however, I begin to warm up to them. Each and every coach rises to rave about the players on his or her team. Never mind if they didn't win all season. Every child is lauded for his or her effort. I begin to like this sports message; it isn't just about winning, after all. The goony speeches start to make sense; it almost seems yogic, this message of giving the sport (life) your all, and not caring about winning (the outcome). Well, of course, they *do* care about winning. But here at the year-end dinner, that's not what it's all about.

When Coach Brinkley rises to ramble on about the track team, I'm already paying attention, but when he begins to talk about Gino, I inch forward in my seat. He's not going to talk about cancer, I say to myself, not here in this room full of several hundred people.

But not only is he talking about cancer, he's talking about Gino's cancer specifically. He's describing how it kept him out of school for months, and how his teammates, classmates, and teachers were so worried, and how the track season started without Gino, and without the real hope of him returning to the sport. He describes how Gino finally returned, how he fought his cancer, how he didn't win his first race back, but how he ran anyway. "I tried to discourage Gino because I was afraid that running might weaken him," the coach admits, "but he insisted, and when he reached the finish line that day, breathless and exhilarated, he cried out triumphantly, 'Six months ago I was battling cancer, and today I'm running track!'"

I know just how Gino felt; just as I felt the other night dancing. It's that sense of wonder and gratitude that arises when life changes so dramatically, when you've stepped so close to the edge and survived. In Gino's case, especially, whose Stage III cancer was critical.

So this sets my tears flowing, and when "Circle of Life" is played and the final slide show is presented, and on the screen above us is image after image of Sam conducting the band, of Gretchen playing volleyball, of Gino running, and of all the other kids living life so fully, well, needless to say, I'm weeping. But I'm not alone. Half the audience is bawling, even some of the dads. As I leave the hall, a rough-hewn football player with tattoos and a pierced ear, pats me on the shoulder. "Hey, Mama," he whispers. "It's *okay* to cry."

Tonight as I drift off to sleep, I consider two lessons I've learned this year. The first, that when you're in the darkness, know that the light will come. We are light and dark, sun and moon, male and female, yin and yang; life is composed of opposites, in a continuing cycle of change.

The second, when you are in the light, don't step back into

the darkness. Live in that light, and breathe it in fully. I've spent so much of my life going over and over the sadness and fear of the past. But we don't need to go there when we're not there. When we are in the light, be here, now.

∞

The writers' group meets tonight at my house. It's cool and breezy outside but we wear our jackets and sit on the deck near the new plum tree. Tonight, we aren't here to talk about writing; we're celebrating the end of my treatments and catching up on our lives. Jessica has been studying to become an interfaith minister and she's also into chanting, so she leads us in a Sanskrit chant of compassion. She offers a few poem/prayers, too, and as she reads aloud I think about how the four of us have been together for nearly six years now, moaning and complaining about our writing careers. But tonight we are just friends, just women who love and care for one another.

As we chant, I glance toward Jess, whose voice is clear and willowy. We close our eyes and imagine light—an unspoken color of our own choosing, a color we will then announce and pass to the woman at our right. Jessica's is blue, Kayla's is white, Amy's is red, and mine is gold. I don't know why I see gold (maybe it's the golden yellow of the solar plexus chakra, the location of personal power), or why we each intuitively choose a different color. I am receiving white light from Kayla and passing gold to Amy.

Jessica offers thanks that we know each other, and asks us to be open to the light. "Receiving from a friend is a gift in itself," she observes. "In receiving light, love and help, we give back the gift of acceptance."

I give each of my friends a tangible gift, too; a polished heart-shaped stone. Jessica's symbolizes clarity, so that she'll continue to define her message; Kayla's is vitality, a reflection of her sparkling, exuberant personality, and Amy's is courage, to deal with three unruly adolescent sons (a bit like mine). Lest anyone think we're a coven of pagan witches or New Age hippies, we conclude our special meeting by gossiping about the latest real estate sales in their pricey, upscale town; we even manage to bitch and moan a bit about writing, just like old times.

I'm grateful that my writer friends have been with me on this journey.

When we first sat down to discuss markets and agents, and critique one another's work, we never foresaw that one cool spring evening in the future we'd be celebrating the end of cancer treatments together. But life is sometimes a mystery penned by a clever, unpredictable muse.

Marathon yoga day. I begin with Jill's class this morning. She recounts the well-known (in spiritual circles, anyway) tale of the snake and the rope. A man comes home at night and spies a mammoth, menacing snake on the ground outside his doorway; he cries out and the neighbors rush over to help him beat it to death. But before they can begin, another neighbor shows up with a lantern; he shines his light on the evil snake, which turns out to be a coiled rope— in the darkness an entirely false reality has been concocted. I've heard this story before, but today it resonates. How silly that we even want to conjure up a snake.

This notion of perspective and illusion also relates to some of the poses we do today. Jill has us crouch on the floor, wrapping our arms through our legs, then rise with arms still wrapped and leg outstretched to a pose she calls Bird of Paradise. You see, it's all how you look at it: I'd be more likely to call this asana Bird of Purgatory. It's not quite Hell, but it sure ain't Heaven. Anyway, I can't do it!

I attempt the difficult Firefly pose, however, and for a few seconds I manage to lift my weight with my hands on two foam blocks and cross my feet in front of me. Even in a class of "no competition" everyone laughs and claps when something like this is accomplished—especially by yours truly.

This afternoon, I return to the center. Natalie has invited me to help test-drive a new teacher along with Jill, a few other teachers, and Natalie herself. The teacher practices Anusura yoga, which incorporates Iyengar's alignment techniques with respect for the inner heart. Part of Anusura's message is one of grace, and the teacher keeps repeating "open to grace" as we practice. I think about this word, this word that has so many meanings for me. The grace of God (the divine bestowing of goodness), my dear Aunt Grace (who survived childhood meningitis and was a corker), Amazing Grace (with its funereal majesty), Sam's pretty friend Grace (who might have been a better match for him than Gretchen), saying grace at the table (which we never do, though I certainly thank the Great Beyond every day for all that I hold dear in life). I think of the word graceful, which I am not but would like to be. Yet maybe I am something even better: grace-full.

Since everyone seems to have a hip issue today, I'm the only one who can come close to the split (otherwise known as Hanuman, or Monkey God Pose) this instructor asks of us, a fact that brings laughter to Jill and Natalie, though the diminutive, soft-spoken teacher doesn't get the joke. It's kind of comical that in a room of yoga teachers, only the cancer survivor student can manage the pose.

When I arrive home Ben is studying for his biology final, and Sam is working on the speech he must give as Salutatorian (he's number two and seems fine with it now). He has a beginning and an end, he says, but nothing in the middle. His task is to write about the past; the Valedictorian covers the future.

"But everything I think of writing," Sam complains, "sounds like the *ending* of the speech."

"That's appropriate," I point out. "After all, the students are ending a chapter of their lives, and so you're just looking back at all the tiny endings along the timeline that have led to this moment. But inherent in every ending is a beginning; the end of one phase is the start of another."

I'm smiling when I leave Sam's room; I've given my son the very lesson his mother needs to hear.

∞

Eloise and I talk on the phone for a long time this morning. Her son will be a senior next year, and she's been following my progress carefully. She's worried, of course, because Jeb is her only child and she'll be retiring from teaching soon. She can't imagine what she'll do when he's gone off to college.

Eloise has learned from me, though, and I'm certain she'll find meaningful ways to occupy her time. She's joined a book club already, and has noticed that when she gets together with other women to talk about books, she always ends up laughing and forgetting her problems for a while. This is why I have my writers' group, my book club, even my wine club. When her parents celebrated their twenty-fifth anniversary, Eloise confides, her mother promised her dad, "The first twenty-five years were yours. The next twenty-five are mine." But they didn't have another twenty-five years together. Why wait for life to happen?

I take a brisk walk after our chat, and when I come home I find that Sam has made himself blueberry pancakes and is just cleaning up the kitchen. The house smells delicious, and a wave of pride and sorrow washes over me. This is the first time my son has ever made himself pancakes for breakfast. This bird is ready to fly.

∞

I miss Jill's class today because I'm scheduled for my six-month follow-up MRI. My niece, Lisa, is visiting from North

Carolina, and she offers to come with me, but Mitch is free and Lisa had prior plans to go into the City with a friend, so I tell her not to worry, I'll be fine. "I'd be fine, even if I had to go solo," I assure her.

Lisa and Mitch exchange glances. "Wow," she says, "you *have* changed."

I guess the new me is still a bit of a novelty around these parts. It's weird to hear *me* say, "Whatever. No problem."

I pop a Xanax when I get to the testing lab. I could rely on my yogic breathing exercises or my new, more optimistic perspective on life, but one never knows how one will feel when one is breast-down on a table with what sounds like a construction team working in one's brain. As it turns out, I'm happy I've taken the pill because it's incredibly hot in the MRI room today and as soon as I'm in place, listening to my Marriage of Figaro CD between the hammering, I do feel rather claustrophobic. But everything is relative, and compared to making my radiation mold this is nada. I just close my eyes, breathe, and pretend I'm meditating. I'm just hanging out here for a bit, face down with my boobs dangling below me. *Chillin'* as Ben would say.

When the test is over, I promise myself that I won't go down the various horror routes in my mind. I'll get the results when I get the results, and they will be what they will be. Yes, I'm chanting positive words to myself, and focusing on all the proactive steps I've taken in the past six months to ensure that this disease will never return, but in reality, once you've had cancer, I don't think it's possible to completely erase the fear of its recurrence. *What if.* Those two horrid words again.

But, let's turn the dial on them. What if I hadn't gone for a mammogram when I did? What if I hadn't found a caring, skilled surgeon? What if I had never practiced yoga? What if I had never met Jill? What if I had never realized how blessed and lucky I am, how blessed and lucky we *all* are to be living on this earth? What if I had spent the rest of my life fearing the future, regretting the past, letting the moments slip by without honoring them? What if, *indeed*, as Eloise always says.

So I will "wait" for my results, but while I'm waiting, I'll practice yoga, meet with my writer friends, get together with the wine club. I'll help Ben study for finals, watch Sam graduate, chat with Aaron when he comes home from work at night, and I'll be as kind as I can to my husband.

What if...I never awakened?

Epilogue: Namaste

I'm feeling rather down, having dropped my niece at the airport. I loved having her here; Mitch says we're like two blue jays chattering. When either my sister or niece come to visit, I realize how good it is to have another woman in the house; we shop, we cook, we talk and talk. It's always hard to say good-bye.

I'm worried, too, about my MRI results. I've vowed not to dwell on the topic, but I can't completely shake my uncertainty. I suppose that from now on even those "routine" tests will never seem quite so routine again.

Rather than sit home, I head for the town pool with a book, settling under a shady maple tree. I flip the pages, but I can't really concentrate. I often meet Anneke under this tree in the late afternoon, but she's not here today. The water looks inviting, but throwing myself in seems brash, and the idea of slipping in slowly doesn't appeal, either.

My cell rings, and I grab for it, thinking it's Lisa, calling to tell me she's safely back in North Carolina. Instead, it's Sam.

"Mom? Your doctor called and said your MRI was fine," he

reports. "I just came in and found the message on the answering machine."

My MRI is fine. I won't need another for six months! Sam has called me at the pool, knowing how much this means to me. My Sam, my sons, such wonder.

I remove my amber necklace and place it gently on my towel, then walk to the edge of the pool. One foot in, then the other, just an instant of hesitation before I plunge into the cold, clear water. Children splash and kick nearby, but I swim past them. I float on my back and close my eyes. With the hot, bright sun beating above, I envision a white light, then a golden light; my body cools and relaxes as gratitude fills my heart.

I think of the trip Lisa and I made to the Metropolitan Museum of Art yesterday. The Met is home to a number of Ganesh statues—my friend, the elephant-headed remover of obstacles. I think of the room of Buddhas and the quiet power they held. As soon as I stepped into that room I felt the silence and peace.

Floating in the cold water, with my eyes closed and the hot golden sun above, I feel that peace again. I am *here, now.*

#

Acknowledgments

So many people have helped me on this journey—some whom I've known for many years, some who are strangers. I can't possibly name them all, but I will do my best. If I leave out a name, for privacy reasons or through neglect—you know who you are, and I thank you.

First, to my family: Mitch Kriegler, and our sons, Aaron, Sam and Ben, for their support and love. And to my mother-in-law, Bertha Kriegler, a powerful yogini herself. Thank you to my wonderful sister, Ruthann Hoffman, my brother-in-law Thomas Hoffman, my brother James Livingston (for all those phone calls!) and to my sister-in-law Carolyn Meyers. Thank you to my beautiful niece Lisa Hoffman and her fiancé Matthew Hickman (for the laughs), and to James and Joan Hoffman and Jason Livingston. Thank you to Amy and Natalie Kriegler, Bob Charla, Chris Paccione, Julianne Paccione, Harold and Maureen Zarember and to all the other members of my loving and exceptional family, with a special nod to Susie Frahm and Thomas Swart. Gratitude to my mother and father, who are within me, for all that they gave me.

Second, thank you to my amazing spiritual sisters: Francine Lipani, Pan DuBois, and Barbara Warner, who are always there for me.

Thank you to Abigail Gary, Maureen Jeffries, and Kim Mendelsohn for their unwavering enthusiasm and encouragement; thanks to all the other members of the GR Book Club, including Leigh Ann Geen, Ellen Dowling, Kathryn Longo and Karen Major. Gratitude also to Lila Corn Rosenweig (for all those ideas!) and Elaine Silverstein.

Of course, thank you Bob and Grace Gynn, Anita and John Viaud, Barbara Valencia, Phyllis Cortese, Sue and Ray Carlton, and Renee and John Czarnecki—you have all given me so much laughter and love.

I would also like to thank, for their support, friendship, caring, advice and/or inspiration: Walter Phelps, Bob Frank, David Markus, Louis and Pilar Cruz, Paul Gary, Abigail Johnson, Dory Streett, William Rosenfeld, Nancy McGurty, Janet Montalbano, Joyce Bendavid, Maryanne Kearney, Kim Lauzon, Ray, Darla, Rayna and Darlayne Addabbo, Debbie Pumo, Patti Dobish, Susan Sands, Maxine Ramey, Milinda Carson, Jean Padovan, Omar Nadeem, and Scott and Kim Liguori. Thanks also to Francis Bonny, William Scribner and Marsha Heller, Geri Koch and Naomi Katz, George and the too soon departed Jane Cochrane, Richard and Barbara Hagen, Elaine Sutin, Mark Rotella, Akalsukh Singh, Jay Bolsom, Dee Andalkar, Elizabeth Shammash, Anayra Calderon, Sandra Varano, Carl Rosenblum, Ron DuBois, Andrejs Jansons, Penni Feiner, Mary Ellen Scherl, Elizabeth Boleman-Herring, Sarah Tomlinson, Desiree Rumbaugh, Reverend Jaganath Carrera, Angela Zito and Dr. Susan Love's Army of Women. My deep appreciation for the writings and spirit of Paramahansa Yogananda.

Thank you to my top-notch physicians at Hackensack University Medical Center who lovingly and professionally touch the lives of cancer patients every single day, and to the caring and extraordinary staff there. Thank you Mary Jane Warden and Robert Alter in particular.

A special thank you to dearest Nancy Siegel and to everyone who studied and taught at that sacred space called Nesheemah.

Namaste, and a heartfelt thank you to Charlotte Stone of Stone Center for Yoga and Health, a remarkable, gentle yogini from whom I have learned so much.

From the depths of my heart, gratitude to Liz Aitken-O'brien, a compassionate and extraordinary woman and teacher.

Thank you to Amy M. Schiffman of Intellectual Property Group for her hard work on my behalf, and for her support and invaluable friendship.

Gratitude to Thomas Ellsworth, Hutch Morton, Julie Morales, Ryan Shaw, Jeannine McHenry, and the fantastic team at Premier Publishing for making my dream of sharing my story come true. A huge thank you to Maria Kuzmiak for her excellent copyediting work and support.

Finally, my deepest thanks to all of my yoga teachers, to the peace-loving world of yoga and to all who share in it.

And, as my mother would say, "Thanks be to God!" and to the Universe, and to the abiding power of love, healing and trust. Namaste.

00562 5313

CPSIA information can be obtained at www.ICGtesting.com
Printed in the USA
BVOW02s1704100414

350025BV00001B/1/P